What in the World is Treatment Resistance in Psychiatry?

(That is, Mental Disorders that Do Not Respond to Treatment)

What in the World is Treatment Resistance in Psychiatry?

(That is, Mental Disorders that Do Not Respond to Treatment)

Written By:
Austin Mardon
Razan Ahmed
Katerina Bavaro
Kendall Caperchion
Jessica Henschel
Hassan Khan
Ruchira Nandasiri
Megha Sharma
Rosalie Sullivan
David Supina
Kelly Wu

Editor:
Stephanie Lazar

Cover Design By:
Josh Harnack

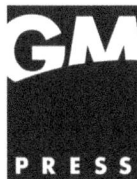

First Printing: 2021

Typeset and Cover Design by Josh Harnack

ISBN: 978-1-77369-249-4

Golden Meteorite Press
103 11919 82 St NW
Edmonton, AB T5B 2W3
www.goldenmeteoritepress.com

Table of Contents

What is the History of Treatment Resistance?

by Jessica Henschel

Introduction

The fields of psychiatry and psychology are relatively young compared to other medical disciplines. The modern era of providing care for the mentally ill began early in the 19th century and the profession did not become scientifically researched and backed until the beginning of the 20th century (Shorter, 1997). Subsequently, the concept of treatment resistant psychiatric illness did not come about until modern treatments (including new therapies and psychopharmacology) of clinical mental disorders were employed starting in the 1950s (Elkis, 2010). Treatment resistant mental illness refers to disorders that do not respond or benefit from medication, psychotherapy, neuromodulatory treatments, and even electroconvulsive therapy (ETC). To better understand how treatment resistance influences individuals and clinicians, it is essential to look at the roots of psychiatry and psychological practice in history.

Mental Illness in the Ancient World

Medicine and psychiatry have their beginnings in ancient times-specifically in the Greek and Islamic worlds. In ancient Greece (12th-9th century BCE), the major authority on medicine was Hippocrates of Cos (460-370 BCE). Hippocrates was well known for his theories on the four humours, which he believed governed the overall wellness of the human body (Conrad et al.,1995). These humours were: phlegm, blood, black bile, and yellow bile. If any of these humours were out of balance, it would cause illness, including disturbances of the mind. Hippocrates believed that there must be a balance of body and mind in order for true health to be obtained. His theories revolved around the idea that the bodily processes, health, and disease can be explained in the same way as other natural phenomena and are independent of any arbitrary, supernatural interference. Therefore, treatment of mental health disorders constituted a strict regimen and lifestyle change. This included exercise, environment, food, and drink to be aligned with the requirements of the humours (Conrad et al., 1995). Hippocrates also strongly believed in the power of the gods to assist with healing of the mind, especially the god of medicine and healing, Asclepius.

Ancient Greek physicians were primarily concerned with psychoses (externalizing disorders such as mood disorders) rather than neuroses (anxiety or depression) (Beck, 2014). Externalizing disorders were outwardly more concerning to not only physicians and healers, but the general public as well. They consider untoward acts in public, delusions, hallucinations, and delirium to all be part of an illness of the brain. There were limited treatment options available to these doctors and any form of pharmaceutical or oral remedy was hardly used. Despite the attempts to help individuals suffering from mental illness, there were those who did not respond- our first look at treatment resistance (Beck, 2014). These individuals were usually marginalized by society and Greek citizens thought that they were possessed by demons or were being punished by the gods. Unfortunately, those with mental illness were often shunned, locked in their homes, and even put to death on rare occasions (Corrigan, 2002). This is part of the stigma and fear that remains to this day about those with mental illness

Psychiatry and care of the mentally ill can also be traced back to ancient Indian and Hindu traditions. The oldest known texts on psychiatric disorders include the Ayurvedic text Charaka Samhita (Scull, 2014). Ayurveda is a tradition of alternative medicine with historical roots in the Indian subcontinent and is still practiced in modern times, although it has been critiqued as a pseudoscience by allopathic doctors, Therapies typically include special diets, remedies, yoga, massage, and medical oils. The Charaka Samhita is a Sanskrit text on Ayurvedic methods and describes ancient theories on the human body, etiology, therapeutics, and symptomatology (Glucklich, 2008). Similarly to Hippocrates' humourism, the Charaka Samhita emphasises that true health comes from a balance of mind, body, and soul. In order to have bodily health, the mind must also be taken care of. The possibility of disease of the mind comes from an imbalance of what Ayurveda calls "tamas" or "rajas" in the mind, which control an individual's emotional and physical reactions (Behere et al., 2013). It was thought that if either tamas or rajas were out of balance, then emotional disturbances would occur that ancient Indians related to psychological illness. Tamas and rajas are also influenced by toxins from the three Doshas- similar idea to the four humours of ancient Greek medicine.

The concept of mental health treatment is referred to as Sattvavajaya therapy in the Charaka Samhita (Behere et al., 2013). To treat mental illness, Ayurvedic practitioners would prescribe certain health regimens, corrective behaviours, and yoga. Sattvavajaya is the method of treatment in which individuals try to bring their intellect (dhi), fortitude (dhrti), and memory (smrti) into a proper condition. The fundamental purpose of Sattvavajaya is the same as modern day psychiatry- removal of the mind from harmful sense-objects and reducing emotional distress (Behere et al., 2013).

Despite these seemingly progressive approaches to treat mental illness as a true medical condition in ancient India, mental illness was also explained in Ayurveda by exogenous factors — supernatural means, primarily surrounding possession by demons that cause insanity or madness (Smith, 2006). It was regarded as a significant affliction and was therefore medicalized early in the tradition in order to treat these disease-producing possessions. As these symptoms were caused from external means, Ayurvedic practitioners often viewed those with mental illness from possession as suffering from "divine origins" (Smith, 2006). Seizures, convulsions, or any signs of epilepsy were generally associated with illness of the mind and thought to be caused by malevolent spirits. Generally, this diagnosis was given when no other physical or Dosha diagnosis could be found for strange behaviours and thoughts. The division between the mind and body is quite clear in demonic possession, as these demons were used as an explanation when individuals do acts that are against social or religious sanctions. As there seems to be an understanding that demons do not always physically inhabit the body but affect the health of the individual, it suggests that that person was vulnerable to or prone to mental illness out of their own doing. People can become influenced by a demon at certain times or when they fail to perform the expected religious rites or sacrifices (Smith, 2006).

Mental Illness in the Middle Ages

As medicine and social sciences began to progress in the middle ages (5th-15th centuries), so did psychiatry and treatment of mental disorders. It is important to preface that in the Western World, Christianity was a large influencing force on medicine and the view of individuals who experienced mental illness (Conrad et al., 1995). As Christianity developed, the New Testament texts on healing and medicine promoted conflicting approaches and attitudes. However, the most prominent belief was that Christ was the healer of the soul and the more the body appeared a mere temporary habitation of an immortal soul, the less it needed to be attended to (Conrad et al., 1995). This had significant implications for mental illness (what they called "madness"), as those suffering from afflictions of the mind/soul were considered sinners or victims of possession. Deviant behaviours were also attributed to poison or other external forces. As a result, the Christian church would perform elaborate rituals and exorcisms to cure the afflicted (Kelly, 2019).

Around this time, religious hospitals and asylums began to pop up. Christ ordered his followers to care for the sick, poor, lonely, and needy- given institutional form by the creation of "deacons" charged with the distribution of alms (giving money or food). St. Basil actually created "a new city" outside the walls of Caesarea where the sick, leprous, and the poor could get medical assistance (Conrad et al., 1995). Before this time, the care of the mentally ill was mostly tasked to the community or the members of the individual's family. The most significant hospital/asylum - more accurately a prison - was Bethlem Royal Hospital in London or as it was commonly referred to, Bedlam (Ruggeri, 2016). Built in the 13th century, Bethlem began as a religious order and was dedicated to St. Mary of Bethlehem. Over time it became a medieval hospital that specialized in helping people who could not care for themselves- particularly those considered "mad" (Ruggeri, 2016). It is well known that the treatment of inmates at Bethlem was poor and even cruel. The living conditions were horrendous and the interior of the building was shabby and not well maintained. Patients were packed into small cells and were living on top of another due to the sheer amount of people who were incarcerated there. Unfortunately, Bethlem became a dumping ground for anyone who was considered deviant or abnormal.

Another notorious part of Bethlem's history were the various experimental psychiatric treatments. Early psychiatrists performed invasive and tortuous therapies on patients (Casale, 2017). One such treatment was called "rotational therapy", where the individual was placed in a chair and suspended from the ceiling. The chair would then be spun at the discretion of the overseeing doctor and was sometimes done more than 100 times a minute. Often, the patient would vomit and experience extreme vertigo. In 1728, James Monro became Bethlem's chief physician/psychiatrist and shifted treatment to focus on surgical technique (Casale, 2017). From this point on, therapies only got worse- one such method was to routinely beat, starve, and drunk patients in ice baths. However, one of the most concerning events at Bethlem was the period of time when they opened their doors to the public to come and view the patients, as if they were zoo animals. Rich Londoners would pay to be able to roam the halls and experience the psychosis and chaos of Bethlem. This was demeaning and humiliating for patients, especially those who were truly suffering from mental illness. Unfortunately, mental disorders were not understood and the general public had a morbid fascination and terror of it (Casale, 2017).

Modernization and Scientific Reform of Psychiatry

The modern era of providing care for the mentally ill did not begin until the 19th century. Public asylums were established in Britain and committees were formed to evaluate misconduct and abuse at private institutions (Clive, 1993). An important change was the Lunacy Act of 1845 that changed the overall treatment of the mentally ill and mandated that they be cared for as patients and receive proper treatment. All across Europe governments were attempting to reform the purpose and maintenance of asylums to avoid mistreatment. In the United States, the building of state asylums began with the passing of a law in 1842 that dictated asylums should exist for those in need. This came hand in hand with new scientific advances in the field of psychiatry. Categories of mental illness were broadened to include mood disorders and disease level delusion and irrationality. The term psychiatry was not actually coined until 1808 by Johann Christian Reil and means "soul/mind healer" in Greek (Schochow & Steger, 2013). As a pioneer of psychiatry - alongside Phillipe Pinel and Jean Etienne Dominique - he vehemently argued for the introduction of public insane asylums and the humane treatment of these individuals who were housed there. He took a comprehensive approach that encompassed psychiatry, psychosomatics, and medical psychology as one entity (Schochow & Steger, 2013).

It was in the 20th century that psychiatry began to take off and be recognized as a true medical discipline. Different perspectives of looking at mental illness were introduced. One individual who significantly influenced the development of psychiatry in this time was Emil Kraepelin (Shorter, 1997). Kraepelin was interested in more comprehensive ideas of psychology and began studying the idea of disease classification for mental disorders. He stated that the differences between mental disorders was biology and this evolved into a new concept of nerves and psychiatry became the model for neurology and neuropsychology (Shorter, 1997). When Kraepelin tried to find the organic causes of mental illness, he began adopting a positivist medicine approach. However, Kraepelin was later criticized for his perspective that schizophrenia was a biological illness even with the absence of detectable anatomical abnormalities.

Beginnings of Treatment Resistance in Psychiatry

It is difficult to pinpoint when exactly the concept of treatment resistance in psychiatry became apparent to psychiatrists and psychologists, as there has always been mental illness that did not respond to therapy. As we have seen, the Hippocratic and Ayurvedic procedures alike did not always produce favourable results. This pattern continued into the time of Bedlam and later psychiatrists. However, the beginnings of treatment resistance research and awareness began with schizophrenia and with the idea that treatment resistance was primarily a lack of response to psychiatric pharmaceuticals (Elkis, 2010). Soon after the discovery of chlorpromazine (one of the very first antipsychotic medications) in 1950, it was seen that a specific group of patients remained symptomatic. Therefore, they were considered resistant to phenothiazines. Since schizophrenia is a life-long, chronic illness, it was a large set back to see that these individuals could not seek reprieve through medication (Elkis, 2010). The first operational definition of treatment resistant schizophrenia was posed in 1988 in the pivotal study that introduced clozapine for treatment of that condition. Based on this definition, treatment resistance in psychiatry is diagnosed when psychotic symptoms persist after failure to respond to two adequate treatment trials with antipsychotics (Elkis, 2010). One of the most important developments in treatment resistance for psychiatry was the introduction of "staging" or classifications of measuring and evaluating the resistance (Fava et al., 2020). Following the introduction of the concept of staging in psychiatry (the detailed process of evaluating where an individual exists on a continuum of their disorder from 0 to stage IV) in 1993, there were different methods to stage the degrees of treatment resistance as well. There are a variety of staging methods that were proposed, but no singular one was deemed more superior. Thase and Rush proposed a 5-stage model where patients were categorized according to the number and class of antidepressants or antipsychotics that failed to have a response, with staging from more common to less common therapies. The Massachusetts General Hospital model of staging considered both the number of failed treatment trials and the intensity of the trials without assigning a hierarchy of antidepressant classes (Fava et al., 2020). Eventually, the Maudsley Staging Method was able to incorporate the number of failed trials and factors considered to be closely related to the psychiatric illness such as duration, severity, treatment failure with pharmaceuticals, use of augmentation, and use of electroconvulsive therapy. At the end of this process, the treatment resistance was scored ranging from 3 to 15.

As treatment resistance was studied further, it was found that resistance tended to develop over the course of a patient's illness (Sheitman & Lieberman, 1998). However, it has been shown that a longer time period of untreated psychosis at the early stages of illness (specifically schizophrenia) is associated with longer remission times, a decreased level of recovery, and a greater chance of relapse. Therefore, a plethora of studies have been dedicated to examining treatment resistance and furthering knowledge of how to identify and manage it. This gives hope for the future of treatment resistant psychiatric disorders and allows patients to live a better and more fulfilling life that is not weighed down by mental illness.

How was Treatment Resistance Discovered?

by Rosalie Sullivan

Treatment Resistance and its Discovery

The concept of Treatment Resistance was first discovered in the 1950s when asylums and mental hospitals became the preferred form of treatment for patients (Fava et al., 2020). Doctors and psychiatrists first began noticing treatment resistant psychiatric disorders when they realized that the patients were failing to respond to treatment (Fava et al., 2020). When antidepressant drugs and medication failed to impact the patient's health and mental well-being, the asylums took notice of it. A diagnosis of Treatment Resistance was then formulated, as doctors and psychiatrists discovered more and more patients whose conditions were not improving with medication (Fava et al., 2020). Treatment resistant psychiatric disorders have been around since the dawn of medicine, but were only truly discovered when modern treatments became popularized. Doctors and psychiatrists only took notice of the psychiatric disorder when antidepressants drugs and other medication were available. There was, however, no one doctor or psychiatrist that discovered Treatment Resistance. The identity of the doctor who first diagnosed a patient with Treatment Resistant is unknown and a mystery. The concept of Treatment Resistance first came about when modern treatments were popularized, but that is all that is known about the psychiatric disorder and its discovery.

Witchcraft and Demonic Possession: The Medieval Perceptions of Mental Health

Throughout history, witchcraft was perceived as a harmful religious practice. It involved the study of maleficia (harmful magic) and diabolism (worship of the Devil) (Russel, 1972). People believed that witches were servants of the Devil, and that they desired chaos and anarchy. Witches were seen as the cause of social disorder, and witch trials were implemented in an attempt to eradicate them and their harmful practices. In reality, witch trials predominantly accused innocent women who were 'senile' and mentally ill (Russel, 1972). Many of the women accused did not actually practice or engage in any form of witchcraft. The women were targeted usually because they were mentally ill or simply an easy target. Women who were old, divorced, sexually promiscuous, or mentally ill were targeted at an unprecedented rate (Russel, 1972). The witch trials were essentially a way for the community to dispose of those who did not fit society's expectations and standards. Those who were mentally ill often did not fit into these standards.

"It was [also] believed that mental illness was caused by demonic possession" (Lumen Learning, 2021), and that the mentally ill needed to be 'exorcised' or disposed of. Mental illnesses were attributed to witchcraft and demonic possession, and those suffering from a mental illness were dehumanized and subjugated to cruel treatment. The behaviour of someone who was mentally ill was often seen "as a sign that a person was possessed by demons" (Lumen Learning, 2021). Abnormal behaviours were associated with demonic possession, and the treatment one would undergo to be 'exorcised' would often kill them (Lumen Learning, 2021).

Over time, however, Europeans slowly began to realize that mental illness was something that existed separate from witchcraft. Witchcraft "ceased to be legally [prosecutable]" and people began to reject the "existence of sorcery and witchcraft" (Russel, 1972). Mental illnesses and disorders were gradually accepted by the medical community, and institutions were put in place to house the mentally ill. Asylums, in particular, became a place where the mentally ill could reside. Instead of undergoing a witch trial because of their mental disorder, they were instead being brought to asylums and other mental hospitals.

The Introduction of Asylums and Mental Hospitals

Asylums and mental hospitals were the very first institutions that were created with the intention of housing the mentally ill (Lumen Learning, 2021). Asylums were implemented, however, for the purpose of "ostracizing [patients] from society rather than treating their disorders"

(Lumen Learning, 2021). The mental hospitals did not actually care about helping their suffering patients, rather, they were only interested in isolating them from the world. Those who were mentally ill were stigmatized and discriminated against, and they were seen as vile affronts to nature. Patients were "kept in windowless dungeons, [they were] beaten, chained to their beds, and [they] had little to no contact with [their] caregivers" (Lumen Learning, 2021). The quality of life in these asylums and mental hospitals were abysmal, and many patients suffered under the deteriorating conditions.

"The first recorded Lunatic Asylum in Europe was the Bethlem Royal Hospital in London" (The Time Chamber, 2017) which was established in 1247. The Bethlem Royal Hospital was designated and founded as a "Priory of the New Order of our Lady of Bethlehem" during the reign of Henry the III (Science Museum, 2018). The asylum's conditions, however, were less than satisfactory, and the hospital was more like a prison than anything else. The Bethlem Royal Hospital, as the first Lunatic Asylum in Europe, set the standard for all future asylums and mental hospitals—a standard that was worryingly low. All asylums and mental hospitals that followed the Bethlem Royal Hospital were similarly dysfunctional. They lacked proper healthcare, and they tortured patients more than they helped them.

In asylums, the use of physical restraints was commonplace and seen as acceptable (Science Museum, 2018). The physical restraints often harmed the patients strapped into them, but they were seen as "a necessary part of mental healthcare" (Science Museum, 2018). Even though the "use of restraints demoralised and brutalised [the patients]" (Science Museum, 2018) it was considered a necessary evil. Physical restraints were needed to 'protect' the patient and others from their "anti-social behaviour" (Science Museum, 2018). The use of physical restraints in mental hospitals, however, "only increased the level of violence in the asylum" (Science Museum, 2018). Patients in mental asylums were not treated with respect or dignity, and they were often dehumanized and treated as if they were nothing but animals. Their mental health issues were demonized, and they were subjugated to discrimination and sometimes even torture. The physical restraints that were forced upon patients was one form of restrictive torture that they had to endure. Sometimes the patients would be forced to wear straight-jackets, at other times they would be chained with steel tight manacles (Science Museum, 2018). If one suffered from a mental illness during this time period, they would be subjugated to all kinds of torture. Physical restraints being just one.

During the late 1700s, however, attitudes toward mental health and asylums began to change. Philippe Pinel, a French physician, argued that patients confined in asylums deserved more humane treatment (Lumen Learning, 2021). The French physician argued that patients would not benefit from being chained up and physically restricted, and he claimed that mental stimulation would only help them. He asserted that the patients' caretakers should converse with them regularly and provide them with genuine human interaction. Philippe Pine's suggestion was then put to the test at La Salpêtrière in Paris in 1795 (Lumen Learning, 2021). Just like how he suggested, however, the patients did benefit from "more humane treatment" (Lumen Learning, 2021). Regular mental stimulation, verbal conversations, and less physical restrictions, greatly benefited the patients at La Salpêtrière, and many patients' mental health improved. Quite a few of the patients being kept at the asylum were even "able to leave the hospital" (Lumen Learning, 2021) after a moderate period of time.

Near the end of the 1700s, William Tuke was another man who advocated for better treatment at asylums and all other mental health institutions. He "founded a private mental institution outside York called The Retreat" (Science Museum, 2018) and he followed in Philippe Pinel's footsteps. William Turke argued that mental health patients deserved to be treated like regular human beings, and he asserted that they should not undergo cruel and unfair treatment. Physical restraints, for example, were deemed unnecessary and unusually cruel by him, and he advocated for better and fair treatment. Later on, William Turke's grandson would continue his work, and they would attempt "to tailor treatment to each patient and [house] patients with similar conditions together" (Science Museum, 2018). Overall, the late 1700s were a time of great change in the mental health community, and the unfair treatment that was used in asylums began to get changed.

Treatment Resistance in Asylums and Mental Hospitals

As the conditions in asylums and mental hospitals improved, Treatment Resistance was discovered and diagnosed. When asylums and mental hospitals' medical care was inadequate, patients were never properly taken care of or diagnosed properly. They were given insufficient treatment, and they were often treated as if they were lesser—as if they were worthless. When asylums and mental hospitals, however, began improving their care and treatment, more and more patients were diagnosed properly (Science Museum, 2018). Patients were treated with more respect and dignity, and more accurate diagnoses and treatment plans were established. The treatment, however, was still not as advanced as treatment today. The patients were also not treated as kindly or amicably as they could have been. Patients were still discriminated against, stigmatized, and often hurt, but it was not as bad as it had been before in the past. Conditions were slowly but surely improving—changing for the better. Patients were being offered more accurate and precise treatment, and medication was more effective.

With the improving conditions, however, doctors and psychiatrists were learning more and more about mental disorders—including Treatment Resistant. Treatment resistant psychiatric disorders became discovered and more well known as more and more patients remained unaffected by treatment. When doctors realized that patients did not "respond to multiple antidepressant treatment trials" (Leckband, 2014), they became curious and confused. The patients were not responding to sufficient doses of medicine, and none of their conditions were improving (Leckband, 2014). Doctors and psychiatrists then slowly began to realize that patients with certain mental disorders could in fact be resistant to medical treatment. Some patients were more resistant to medical treatment and antidepressant drugs than others.

The doctors and psychiatrists then began researching Treatment Resistance, gathering more information on it, creating studies, testing patients, and they came to some interesting conclusions. They discovered that "treatment resistance [could] be due to unrecognized exogenous anxiogenic factors (eg, caffeine overuse, sleep deprivation, use of alcohol or marijuana) or an incorrect diagnosis (eg, atypical bipolar illness, occult substance abuse, attention deficit-hyperactivity disorder)" (Roy-Byrne, 2015). To ensure that patients would respond to treatment and antidepressant drugs properly, doctors and psychiatrists had to focus more time and effort on diagnosing patients properly. If a patient was misdiagnosed, the treatment plan put in place for them would not be as effective. Doctors and psychiatrists then also began focusing on eliminating exogenous anxiogenic factors that could negatively impact patients (Roy-Byrne, 2015). This included removing caffeine from their diets and establishing set bed-times. Once these changes were implemented, however, the patients' conditions did in fact improve considerably. More and more patients were sufficiently responding to treatment, and the antidepressant drugs were significantly more effective.

The discovery of Treatment Resistance in asylums and mental hospitals had been quite a shock to the medical community, but the doctors and psychiatrists were slowly but surely discovering a solution to the psychiatric disorder. Even though Treatment Resistance was not entirely curable, treatment for the psychiatric disorder was improving with every passing day (Demyttenaere, 2019). Treatment resistance was defined as a " difficult to treat" (Demyttenaere, 2019) psychiatric disorder, but the asylums and mental hospitals were discovering more effective modes of treatment.

Over time, however, doctors and psychiatrists then slowly began to realize that "treatment should focus on combining effective medications and cognitive behavioral therapy" (Roy-Byrne, 2015) to have the largest impact possible on the patient. Deploying this kind of treatment would benefit the patient greatly—no matter what mental disorder they were affected by. Patients who suffered from Treatment Resistance were often either schizophrenic, depressed, had PTSD (Post Traumatic Stress Disorder), or they possessed some kind of anxiety disorder (Demyttenaere, 2019). All of these mental disorders' coinciding Treatment Resistance could be properly treated with the above mentioned method.

Deinstitualization of Asylums and Mental Hospitals: Moving Towards Modern Day Treatment

With the deinstitutionalization of asylums and mental hospitals, medical care of patients moved from a professional environment to a personal and familial one. Asylums and mental hospitals were closed and shut down, and patients were made to return to their previous homes. The movement would "return those suffering from mental illnesses to their families and their communities" (D'Antonio, 2021). It was decided that the best way to care for patients was to have their families and loved ones take care of them—rather than a hospital (Fakhoury et al., 2007). Hospital care was seen as cold and distant, and many studies were coming to the conclusion that that kind of environment was not beneficial for patients. Patients would make greater strides in their recovery if they were surrounded by their family and friends, not complete strangers—not doctors and psychiatrists (Fakhoury et al., 2007).

The deinstitutionalization of asylums and mental hospitals was also partly motivated because of the development of drug therapies (Fakhoury et al., 2007). Drugs could now be taken in a much more easier and refined manner, and home treatment became possible. Deinstitutionalizing asylums and mental hospitals would also save money for the government which funded these hospitals, and it would re-establish familial bonds between patients and family members (Fakhoury et al., 2007).

Studies, at the time, argued that the deinstitutionalization movement would only benefit those suffering from mental illnesses. There were, however, consequences to this movement. Deinstitutionalization meant that patients who lacked social support would often end up homeless (Fakhoury et al., 2007). These patients did not have families, homes, friends, or communities to return to. When the hospitals were shut down, they were essentially thrown out onto the streets. This created an issue of homelessness. With the deinstitutionalization of asylums and mental hospitals, some patients also began receiving worse treatment and care than before (Fakhoury et al., 2007). They could not afford the medical care and treatment they needed. This caused those suffering from mental illnesses to experience a decline in their health. The belief that one should be cared for by their family and community caused many issues in this way.

Another problem that arose with the deinstitutionalization of asylums and mental hospitals was the issue of transinstitutionalization. Transinstitutionalization is the experience where one patient is moved from one institution to another (Fakhoury et al., 2007). Many patients suffering from mental illnesses were moved from an asylum to a prison. Once the asylums and mental hospitals were shut down, some of the patients were not receiving adequate care and treatment. The result of them not getting this treatment led them to experience conflict with the law (Fakhoury et al., 2007). Since they were not taking their medication or receiving proper care, the police often had to get involved, as their behaviour would often go against the law (Fakhoury et al., 2007). The deinstitutionalization of asylums and mental hospitals created the issue of transinstitutionalization in this way.

With the deinstitutionalization of asylums and mental hospitals, however, medicine and medical practices continued to progress and move towards modern day treatment. By the time the early 2000s rolled around, there was "an exponential increase in papers on treatment resistant psychiatric disorders" (Demyttenaere, 2019). Different mental disorders were becoming more well known, and a deeper understanding of Treatment Resistance and what was needed for a diagnosis had "increased to a considerable degree" (Fava et al., 2020). Treatment Resistance was no longer something that received barely any recognition, it was a diagnosable psychiatric disorder. Modern medicine and drug therapies allowed for Treatment Resistance to become more easily recognizable, and the disorder will most likely become more well known and recognized as medicine continues to advance.

Conclusion

In conclusion, Treatment Resistance was first discovered in the 1950s when asylums and mental hospitals began offering patients more forms of treatment and medicine. Only when drug therapies and antidepressant drugs became popularized, did doctors and psychiatrists begin to realize that some patients were resistant to treatment more than others. Treatment Resistance had existed since the invention of medicine, but it only became diagnosable during the era of mental hospitals. Asylums and mental hospitals were only able to come about, however, thanks to the witch hunts and trials. For most of history, mental illnesses and disorders were seen as the cause of witchcraft—the cause of demonic possession. If a person was mentally ill, or they just existed outside of society's norms, they were ostracized and deemed a witch. When society began to realize that these people were mentally ill and not witches, however, asylums and mental hospitals began to get funded. The asylums used cruel and unusual treatment for their patients, and the mental hospitals were more like a prison than anything else. They used physical restraints on their patients, and the conditions within the hospitals often worsened the patient's condition. Eventually, however, the care and treatment provided in asylums and mental hospitals did begin to change for the better, but it was still far from ideal. As the conditions in asylums and mental hospitals began to improve, however, more studies and research about Treatment Resistance began to form. Treatment Resistance became a diagnosable psychiatric disorder, and its discovery was made in these mental institutions. Different forms of treatment for the psychiatric disorder were discovered, and Treatment Resistance became more well known. Eventually, however, asylums and mental hospitals were closed and shut down for the benefit of the patients. There were, however, a variety of consequences to the deinstitutionalization of mental hospitals as well. Yet in the end, the deinstitutionalization of mental hospitals allowed for society to further progress forward. New drug therapies and forms of treatment came out, and Treatment Resistance became more widely known in the 2000s. As medicine continues to progress in the future, Treatment Resistance is expected to become more well known and understood as well.

What is the Impact of Treatment Resistance?

Macro scale Impact

by Hassan Khan

Introduction

Treatment-resistant disorders include many types of disorders such as depression, anxiety, bipolar disorder, addictions, and schizophrenia (Amen Clinics, n.d.). For example, treatment-resistant depression is a term used in psychiatry to describe a patient who suffers from MDD (Major Depressive Disorder) and is unable to respond to antidepressant drugs (Fava, 2003). As a whole, patients affected by any of these disorders are unable to respond to treatment and can be impacted in a very negative way. Some of those implications are found on a macroscale including healthcare institutions, economic impact, livelihood/quality of life, lethality of the disorders (suicide), and impact on taxpayers. All of these situations add up to make up a bigger picture of the problem behind treatment resistance. These implications are sometimes left unseen and can lead to a spiral of darkness for these patients. It is therefore important to understand what these implications are and how it can affect different people/situations, so that these disorders are brought to the spotlight and are not left in the dark.

Economic Constraints of Treatment-Resistant Depression

The economic burden of treatment-resistant disorders, specifically mood disorders is huge (Demyttenaere & Duppen, 2018). It was reported that mood disorders account for the highest costs for neurological or psychiatric disorders in Europe ($113.4 billion euros) (Demyttenaere & Duppen, 2018). The direct costs are accounted for

37% related to treatment, but indirect costs amounted to 63% for absenteeism or suicide (Demyttenaere & Duppen, 2018). According to recent data, the average cost of mood disorders in the U.S. (United States) increased by 21.5% from 2005 to 2010 (173 billion to 210 billion dollars) (Demyttenaere & Duppen, 2018). The direct costs are accounted for 45% related to treatment, but indirect costs amounted to 60% for suicide related costs (Demyttenaere & Duppen, 2018). For treatment-resistant depression, however, the costs are much higher resulting in more hospitalizations and outpatient visits (Demyttenaere & Duppen, 2018). A recent U.S. study indicated that the direct annual cost of treatment-resistant depression was 40% higher than the cost of non-treatment-resistant depression (Demyttenaere & Duppen, 2018). This was also correlated with the severity of the disorder, with higher severity equalling about 590 dollars increase in annual costs (Demyttenaere & Duppen, 2018).

Health Care Utilization & Costs of Treatment-Resistant Depression

More than 20% of depression patients fail to respond readily to antidepressant treatment trials (Crown et al., 2002). With respect to this, not a lot is known about the health care costs of patients with treatment-resistant depression (Crown et al., 2002). Based on data from the MarketScan Research Database, from Cambridge, Massachusetts, an analysis was conducted to learn more about the health care utilization costs associated with treatment-resistant patients suffering from depression (Crown et al., 2002). There were two groups included in this study, one being the treatment-resistant group and the other being, the comparison group (comprising individuals who responded to treatment) (Crown et al., 2002).

The results showed that treatment-resistant patients were more likely to be diagnosed with a bipolar disorder than the comparison group (Crown et al., 2002). A substantial number of these treatment-resistant patients were hospitalized (twice as likely) due to depression and rarely received outpatient care (Crown et al., 2002). The treatment-resistant group took more medication including antidepressants (1.4 to 3 times) than the comparison group (Crown et al., 2002). Patients in the treatment-resistant group that were hospitalized had about 6 times more medical costs than the individuals successfully responding to treatment ($42,344 vs. $6512) (Crown et al., 2002). Moreover, hospitalized treatment-resistant individuals receiving depression-related care had 19 times the costs of control individuals (Crown et al., 2002). These findings reveal that treatment-related depression has much higher hospitalizations and costs than those responding to treatment (Crown et al., 2002).

In Brazil, the impact of treatment-resistant depression is unknown, although it marks a heavy social impact (Lepine et al., 2012). A study looked at 212 patients diagnosed with 90 of them having treatment-resistant depression and 122 did not have treatment-resistant depression (Lepine et al., 2012). The study gathered information on hospitalizations, medical visits, and procedures (Lepine et al., 2012). Researchers found that treatment-resistant patients were using a significant amount of resources from the psychiatric department, as compared to the non-treatment-resistant group (Lepine et al., 2012). Similar to the previous study mentioned, treatment-resistant patients were more likely to be hospitalized (Lepine et al., 2012). They had much higher costs, about 81.5% annual costs compared to the control group (Lepine et al., 2012).

Social Impact of Treatment-Resistant Depression

In Europe, a study was conducted in five countries (Germany, France, Spain, Italy, and the United Kingdom) to examine the social burden of treatment-resistant depression (Jaffe et al., 2019). About 53,000 patients were looked at initially, after which 2700 and 600 patients were found with treatment-resistant and non-treatment-resistant depression respectively (Jaffe et al., 2019). The results showed that the treatment group and control group were experiencing a decrease in their quality of life, lower physical and mental health, and increased work/activity impairment risk (Jaffe et al., 2019). Treatment-resistant patients were also utilizing their healthcare options (healthcare visits) more than the non-treatment-resistant group (Jaffe et al., 2019). Their emergency visits were also higher than the comparison group (Jaffe et al., 2019). Individuals with MDD were typically younger and female, and less likely to possess a university-level degree or be married (Jaffe et al., 2019). In the general population, individuals were more likely to exercise and consisted of a few non-smokers (Jaffe et al., 2019). Also, those with MDD had cases of chronic heart failure, anemia, diabetes, arrhythmia,

hypertension, arthritis compared to non-MDD patients
(Jaffe et al., 2019).

Treatment-resistant patients showed varying depression
characteristics compared to non-treatment-resistant patients (Jaffe
et al., 2019). They displayed a longer average time since depression
diagnosis as in 12.9 years compared to 10.0 years for the non-
treatment-resistant group (Jaffe et al., 2019). In addition, Jaffe and
colleagues (2019) reported that the treatment-resistant patients'
family members also suffered from anxiety, depression and suicide.
The treatment-resistant patients also took a lot of antidepressants,
antipsychotics, and norepinephrine-dopamine reuptake inhibitors
(Jaffe et al., 2019).

According to the study, hospitalization costs were the largest
contributor of financial burden among other costs with increasing
treatment resistance (Jaffe et al., 2019).

A study was conducted through the PubMed database (from 1996 to
2013) by gathering all relevant articles related to treatment-resistant
depression and its impacts in the U.S (Mrazek et al., 2014). On a scale
of 0 to 1, the quality of life was measured, with 0 representing death
and 1 representing good health (Mrazek et al., 2014). The scores were
relatively low for patients with MDD (0.120 to 0.552) and 0.126 to 0.417
for patients who did not respond to treatment (Mrazek et al., 2014). The
quality of life score declined up to .12 quality of life units if negative
effects followed (Mrazek et al., 2014). Those with treatment-resistant
depression were visiting the medical facility more frequently than those
responding to treatment (Mrazek et al., 2014). About 52% of patients
with treatment-resistant depression were hospitalized over their
lifetimes (Mrazek et al., 2014). According to 2012 US statistics, 16 million
people in the US had M.D.D., and assuming 12% were nonresponsive
to treatment, 1.9 million adults had treatment-resistant depression
(Mrazek et al., 2014). The estimated total cost of treatment for this
population was estimated at 38 billion dollars (Mrazek et al., 2014).
However, another study stated that the true percentage of treatment-
resistant depression patients is around 20% (Mrazek et al., 2014). With
that number, the treatment cost could be around 64 billion dollars a
year increasing the societal burden (Mrazek et al., 2014). The burden
of treatment-resistant depression is comparable to that of cancer and

diabetes, yet depression gets only 15th place among conditions that receive research funding (Mrazek et al., 2014).

For caregivers, it is important to know that there are economic and social challenges associated with caring for a treatment-resistant patient (Demyttenaere & Duppen, 2018). Many of them have to deal with dependence and fear of suicide issues for treatment-resistant patients (Demyttenaere & Duppen, 2018). Caregivers are also known to have a high caseload with 34% of them reported to have some type of psychiatric illness (Demyttenaere & Duppen, 2018). There is also a stigma associated with having a mental illness which leads to more depressive symptoms for caregivers (Demyttenaere & Duppen, 2018). This in turn complicates their situation when caring for a treatment-resistant patient (Demyttenaere & Duppen, 2018).

Despite all these negative impacts of treatment-resistant depression, the actual burden is underestimated due to the limited number of studies on criminality, use of social services, and quality of life burden caused to families and caregivers (Mrazek et al., 2014).

Treatment-Resistant Schizophrenia & Impacts

Schizophrenia is described as a mental disorder that affects the way individuals view reality (abnormally) (Correll et al., 2019). It is treated with available antipsychotics, however positive symptoms are still seen in patients even after taking medication (Correll et al., 2019). It was found that a response rate of 50% was common after one year of antipsychotic medication (Correll et al., 2019). Treatment-resistant schizophrenia is described as having positive symptoms, but being non-responsive to two or more antipsychotic treatments normal in duration (Correll et al., 2019). It is known to have serious impacts on one's health and career as well as devastating economic impacts on families and individuals suffering from schizophrenia (Correll et al., 2019). Researchers have noted that, though drug costs are low for this type of treatment resistance syndrome, hospitalization and health resource utilization is significantly higher than in non-treatment-resistant schizophrenic patients (Correll et al., 2019).

In the U.S., a study was conducted as a survey to 204 psychiatrists from February 12th, 2017 to March 16th, 2017 (Correll et al., 2019).

They reported that in the last 6 months of their career, the number of schizophrenic patients were around 179 to 229 individuals, in which almost 30% had treatment-resistant schizophrenia (Correll et al., 2019). There were multiple risk factors associated with treatment-resistant schizophrenic patients (more common in them) such as hypertension, insomnia, obesity, and depression (Correll et al., 2019). These symptoms were more severe and occurred more frequently in schizophrenic patients than non-treatment-resistant schizophrenic patients (Correll et al., 2019). According to the psychiatrists, hallucinations and delusions were the most detrimental (get rid of as soon as possible) to both treatment-resistant schizophrenic patients and the control group (Correll et al., 2019). In treatment-resistant schizophrenic patients that displayed the symptoms mentioned above, there was a severe impact on their work life, personal and other relationships, self care, and disturbing behaviour (Correll et al., 2019). They are also at an increased risk of homelessness, suicide, unemployment, substance abuse, and imprisonment (Brain et al., 2018). Treatment-resistant patients are also more likely to rely on caregivers for easy access to transportation, managing finances, housework, and meals (Brain et al., 2018). Psychiatrists were less satisfied with treatment-resistant patients than non-treatment-resistant individuals on progress of symptoms and quality of life (Correll et al., 2019).

In the U.S., about 27 caregivers caring for treatment-schizophrenic patients participated in a study across 8 focus groups (across the states) (Brain et al., 2018). Most patients were diagnosed with schizophrenia for 18 years and some were diagnosed for 10 years (Brain et al., 2018). Several caregivers stated that the patients had adversely impacted their social and mental lives (Brain et al., 2018). One of them described their experience saying, "I think we go out a little less because he is so hard to get out of the house...So we don't go out as much as I would like to. And we certainly don't go to as many public places that I would like to. I used to really enjoy going out and having friends. But it just became such an issue because when I got home, he didn't understand where I was and he would get so paranoid." (Brain et al., 2018). Some also mentioned that their family and romantic relationships were negatively impacted as well (Brain et al., 2018). A few caregivers (22%) mentioned they were taking antidepressants to cope with the situation of being with someone with treatment-resistant schizophrenia (Brain et al., 2018). One of them stated, "Honestly, I had to start taking medication

for depression, too. It just got to be a little too much."
(Brain et al., 2018).

Some caregivers noted their physical health was constantly at risk with sleep problems and lack of self care (Brain et al., 2018). The overall stress of caring for a treatment-resistant patient led to these problems (Brain et al., 2018). Over 78% of caregivers also spoke about the negative impacts on their finances, professional opportunities, employment, and being able to travel as a result of this job (Brain et al., 2018). The demands made them spend less time with themselves/others and take on less jobs to try and get a breath of fresh air (Brain et al., 2018). The overall research shows that caregivers are being negatively affected caring for treatment-resistant schizophrenic patients
(Brain et al., 2018).

Conclusion

It is evident that treatment-resistant disorders make a significant impact on the world as a whole, whether it be economically or socially. Many types of mental disorders are classified as treatment-resistant disorders, which include depression, anxiety, bipolar disorder, addictions, and schizophrenia (Amen Clinics, n.d.). In psychiatry, for example, treatment-resistant depression refers to MDD symptoms which do not respond well to antidepressant treatments (Fava, 2003). Treatment-resistant schizophrenia refers to individuals suffering from an abnormal state of mind and not responding to treatment. It is clear from this chapter that patients affected by any of these disorders are unable to respond to treatment and can be impacted in a very negative way. All of these factors come together to form a bigger picture of the problem behind treatment resistance. The implications of such situations are often masked up and can lead to a spiral of despair for patients. This chapter emphasizes what these implications are and how it can affect different people/situations, so it will help bring their attention to the spotlight and will not leave them in the dark. There is hope for many patients suffering from treatment-resistant disorders with a huge amount of research dedicated to treatment discoveries. Nevertheless, there is still a lot that needs to be done and the next chapter will explore why understanding the impacts of treatment-resistant disorders is so important.

Why is it Important to Study Treatment Resistance?

by Ruchira Nandasiri

Introduction

In general, psychiatric disorders include obsessive compulsive, panic, and anxiety Disorders alongside social phobia (Bystritsky, 2006). These disorders have gained very little attention and yet been inadequately understood, understudied and treated compared to other psychiatric syndromes including mood or psychotic disorders (Bystritsky, 2006). Further, it was reported that roughly one out of three people would attain some sort of anxiety disorder sometime at some point in during their lifespan (Bystritsky, 2006). It was further reported that the costs associated with the treatment resistance (TR) is much higher (40% to 50%) than that of non-resistant depression (Rizvi et al., 2014). Currently, there is no direct definition for the TR, however, if a person fails to respond to 2 or more adequate trials of different classes of antidepressants it is said that person is associated with TR (Souery et al., 1999). This is further closely connected with retrieving the person's medication history. Thus, patients with TR are required to obtain multiple medications with provisions to health care facilities (Shelton et al., 2010). Often the treatments include multiple strategies of combined antidepressants, neurostimulation therapies, and electroconvulsive therapies such as repetitive transcranial magnetic stimulations, deep brain stimulations (Rizvi et al., 2011; Shelton et al., 2010).

However, it was reported that patients with TR come-across many side effects in central nervous, gastrointestinal, cardiovascular systems in addition to weight gain and sexual dysfunction (Rizvi et al., 2014). In comparison to other mental health conditions where cost is measured comprehensively by disability and inpatient care in TR patients shows lower productivity and quality of life over the period of time (Bystritsky, 2006). Moreover, it was reported that in the US the costs associated with the anxiety disorders are over 42 billion USD per year which exceeds the total costs correlated with stroke and cardiovascular disorders (Bystritsky, 2006). A recent study conducted by Rizvi et al. (2014) showed that provinces including British Columbia, Manitoba and Ontario have comparatively higher number of TR patients than the national average of 21% (Figure 1). Determining the stereotypes of TR (melancholic, psychotic, atypical, and seasonal) is important in terms of evaluation and management since the response to different subtypes could be variable (Fornaro & Giosuè, 2010).

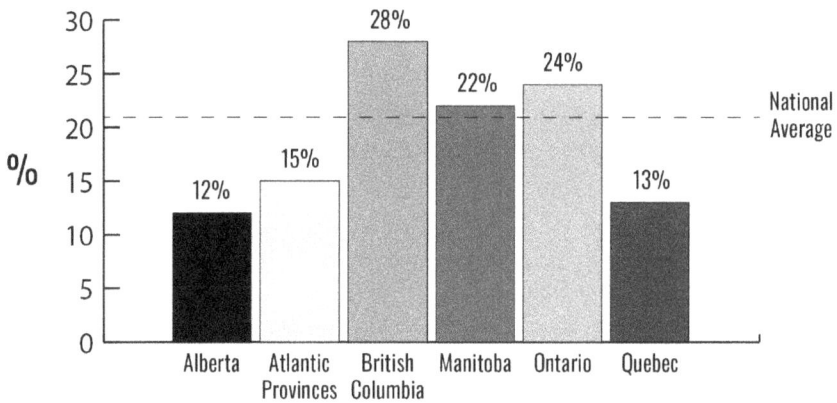

Figure 1: Prevalence of treatment-resistant depression across Canada (Rizvi et al., 2014)

Age and Treatment-resistant (TR)

Age at the commencement of psychosis is generally stated as the age at which first treatment was administered or the age where the symptoms triggered a considerable impairment (Legge et al., 2020). In their study Legge et al. (2020) stated that the risk of TR is not limited to the early onset as previously reported but remained to decrease through adulthood. Their statistical analysis indicated that positive predictive value for TR increased from 0.51 to 0.92 for the individuals who are in the age category of 16 to 41 years of age (Legge et al., 2020). In a different format of a study conducted by Rizvi et al. (2014) reported that higher age groups (50) compared to patients with lower age (47) had greater work impairment compared to non–TR patients indicating the importance of age as a determining factor.

Furthermore, Souery et al. (2006) also reported that early age of onset (<18 years) 1.7% (p<0.009) had a recurrent association with TR. This was further validated by Meltzer et al. (1997) indicating the age at onset of TR is considerably lower than in the non-TR patients. Meltzer et al. (1997) further reported that TR patients would express slight motor behavioural and cognitive abnormalities compared to their siblings and friends during infant and adolescence stages. The authors have further reported that the IQ level of the TR patients are comparatively 5-10 points lower than of the general population. Therefore, the treatment strategies should focus on restoring the intellectual and social potential of the individuals before they attain their early adulthood.

Orientation of Sex on Treatment Resistance (TR)

According to the World Health Organization (WHO), it is reported that around 5-10% of the population at a given time would suffer from many clusters of depression whereas risk of developing a mental disorder is around 10-20% in the females and slightly lower in the male population. Furthermore, another study conducted by Hirschfeld & Weissman (2002) reported that MDD is more common in women than men and often begins during young adulthood. This was further confirmed by Meltzer et al. (1997) in their study reporting women have a significantly later onset of TR than men compared to the non-TR patients. Moreover, in another study conducted by Kubitz et al. (2013) reported that over 30% of the TR patients had complications including joint pain, anxiety, fatigue, migraines whereas non-TR patients only experienced joint pain. Moreover, the prevalence of these comorbid conditions was more prominent in women than the men. On the contrary, a five-year follow-up study conducted by Lally et al. (2016) reported that the relationship among the first contact of the mental health services prior to the age of 20 had a positive relationship among males of Black ethnicity.

Gene Environment Interaction and Treatment-resistance (TR)

Genes has a key important factor on mediation of TR. It is widely reported that the rate of transcription depends on the transporter mechanism whereas shorter allele (s) exhibit lower efficiency than the longer allele (l) (Plakun, 2012). Caspi et al. (2003) in their study reported that patients containing homozygous short alleles (ss) have a higher tendency towards developing mental disorders in response to stress and childhood abuse compared to the patients containing homozygous long alleles (ll). The authors further suggested that apart from the genes, the environment also plays an important role in mediating the mental disorders (Caspi et al., 2003). In addition, Karg et al. (2011) further confirmed that short allele of the serotonin transporter had a higher risk associated with mental stress (p = 0.00002) from a meta-analysis of 54 subjects.

Non-communicable Diseases and Treatment-resistance (TR)

Further analysis indicated that both weight and the body mass index (BMI) of the patients are very closely associated with TR whereas, higher BMI (28.3 kg/m2) compared to lower (26.3 kg/m2) was highly associated with TR (60.1% and 44.8%, respectively) (Rizvi et al., 2014). Moreover, it was reported that patients on lipid-lowering, hypoglycemic and anti-inflammatory drugs have higher risk associated with TR than the other patients (Rizvi et al., 2014). Additionally, it was also reported that patients suffering from cardiovascular diseases, AIDS, cancer, and neurological disorders have relatively higher prevalence towards major depressive disorder (MDD) which initiate TR (Hirschfeld & Weissman, 2002). In another study conducted by Ivanova et al. (2010) stated that TR-patients showed an upsurge in osteoarthritis (5.6%), chronic pain (23.2%) and fibromyalgia (6.4%) compared to the non-TR patients (4.2%, 14.5% and 3.0%) correspondingly.

Social Function, Alcohol and Drug Abuse on Treatment Resistance (TR)

Even though there are numerous clinical and socio-demographic factors that are closely connected with the prevalence of TR it was reported that major two factors including, challenges to adhere to prescribed medication and level of tolerance of the patients accounts for more than half the cases (Nemeroff, 2007). The statistics from the National Alliance of the Mentally Ill indicates that around 15-25% of the schizophrenia patients with TR are unemployed in the US indicating the socio-economic impact on the society. Further, it was reported that over 50% of all schizophrenic patients would fall back to active state in each year due to their limitations of adherence to prescribed medication.

In their study Legge et al. (2020) further illustrated that capability to commence, terminate, or to maintain social relationships prior to psychotic symptoms were closely connected with TR. The multivariate regression analysis further found that lower premorbid IQ levels were closely associated with the increased risk of TR (Legge et al., 2020). In another study by Souery et al. (2006) reported among the psychiatric co-morbidities 3.2% (p<0.001) was on panic disorders, 2.1% (p<0.008) was on social phobia and 2.6 (p<0.001) was on other anxiety disorders indicating the importance of social function on TR. Furthermore, Kendler et al. (2000) reported that childhood sexual abuse was positively connected with many psychiatric and substance use disorders which poses higher TR. Furthermore, the higher treatment costs associated with TR direct towards a loss of economic productivity thereby reducing the quality of life of the people (Plakun, 2012). Additionally, both alcohol and drug abuse play a major role in TR and was shown that alcohol dependency was closely connected with MDD. It was reported that the use of alcohol to reduce anxiety could influence the interactive strategies which may impart an important role in perceiving the corrective actions (Bystritsky, 2006). Furthermore, the substance abuse including alcohol consumption may also impact the adherence to the compliance of medications however, yet there is limited competence to control such measures (Meltzer et al., 1997).

In recent times much emphasis was applied towards managing the common forms of mental stress including TR by engaging health and social care professions, public health agencies, local government, schools, and employers (Bhui, 2017). Social isolation, poverty, unsecured working conditions, unsafe early childhood conditions are major socio-demographic conditions associated with the onset of TR. Thus, it was evident that with greater public engagement with the use of socially embedded, caring, and humane tools improved mental health can be achieved in a shorter time (Bhui, 2017).

Medication, Costs, and Treatment-resistance (TR)

Clinicians and researchers lean towards prescribing lower doses of antidepressants over the time to overcome the obstacles and to minimize the adverse effects (Pandarakalam, 2018). Most common and physician prescribed medications to treat anxiety disorders include selective serotonin reuptake inhibitors (SSRIs) (Roy-Byrne et al., 1998).

However, if the patients are unresponsive to the SSRIs, another class of medication namely serotonin norepinephrine reuptake inhibitors (SNRIs) or tricyclic antidepressants will be administered to treat the disorder (Bystritsky, 2006). Alongside with serotonin containing medications, benzodiazepines are also applied for treating the patients. However, the use of these medications are limited due to its tolerance and dependency (Klein, 2002). The only medication proved to be effective in mediation of TR was clozapine (Leucht et al., 2009).

Apart from the oral medications other types of treatments including cognitive-behavioral treatments are applied widely to treat the anxiety disorders with a success rate of 60-90% (Barlow et al., 2020). Thus, a considerable number of people would still have a lower response towards the cognitive-behavioral treatments which may have an impact on the treatment strategies. Hence, the impact of medication in treating anxiety disorders and TR is still yet to be understood completely. In another note, Katon (1986) found that it is important to oversee the changes continuously in the patients who are admitted to the primary care for a short period of time with a higher oral dosage of SSRIs to determine an adequate response. Further, elsewhere it is reported that switching to an antidepressant with a different mechanism of action would provide a more impressive response rate compared to a one antidepressant to another one in the same class (Pandarakalam, 2018). Multiple medications to treat TR has its own advantages and disadvantages. It was reported that dual antidepressants may contain drug interactions with lower efficacy rates (70%) whereas single drug administrations may have much lower efficacy rates and may have resistance towards the therapeutics (Pandarakalam, 2018). However, it is reported that certain factors including family history, side-effects profile, overdose safety, multiple drug interactions, availability and associated costs would play an important role in selecting certain medications (Unützer & Park, 2012).

In a study conducted by Kubitz et al. (2013) reported that nearly 80% of the non-TR patients only consumed a one line of treatment whereas over 75% of the TR patients utilized no less than four lines of treatments including various classes of antidepressants, combined therapies with recurrent treatments. Apparently, these combined therapies are repeatedly linked with higher medical costs, physician visits, pharmacy and other claims which are about 2.7 to 5.8 times higher than the non-

TR patients (Kubitz et al., 2013). Moreover, TR-patients had higher rate of hospitalizations (0.06), pharmacy claims (7.48), office visits (1.54) and lab visits (0.87) in comparison to non-TR (0.04, 5.15, 1.04, and 0.71 respectively indicating the higher medical costs related to TR (Kubitz et al., 2013). Furthermore, Crown et al. (2002) in their 5-year period of study reported that the overall medical costs of the TR patients ($42,344) was six times higher than the non-TR patients ($6512). Also, the total annual costs of the TR patients ($28,001 for inpatients; $3699 for outpatients) was significantly higher than of non-TR patients ($1455). In addition to the medical related direct costs, it was reported that both the TR patients and their family members had a significant increase in indirect costs including the lower productivity and loss of work (Nemeroff, 2007). Furthermore, the World Health Organization (WHO) and World Bank Global Burden of Disease Study (WBGBDS) in their 2001 report stated that unipolar major depressive disorder alone contributed for over 10% of the global yield whereas neuropsychiatric disorders combined accounted for over 30% of the global yield.

Conclusion

In conclusion, we could state that up-to-date treatment resistance has gained very less attention due to the lack of data and its difficulties in identifying the underlying conditions associated with TR. Further, the emotional distress and mental health problems are not yet considered as serious types of illnesses and studied as a part of everyday life. Tough social experiences, relationship issues, sudden loss of loved ones, and unexpected traumatic events often account for the leading causes of TR. Current treatment techniques to mediate TR is solely dependent on oral medications and often one or more drugs was used. However, lower efficacies associated with oral medications limits the treatment ability and warrants frequent doctor visits. Hence, combined treatment techniques have gained much attention in recent times in treating TR patients. However, these combined treatment techniques are related to a higher number of prescriptive medications and associated costs which may impose further financial stress on the TR patients. Hence, the identification of the symptoms related to TR at early stages of the life before they reach adulthood would impart possible benefits in medical associated costs at their latter part of the life. Furthermore, a treatment method which has a higher efficacy rate, with lower medical associated costs would certainly have a positive impact towards the patients suffering from TR. However, due to the lower progress in the mental health research field the answers to such questions are yet at the horizon.

What is Treatment Resistance?

by Kelly Wu

Introduction

The importance of mental health has steadily and significantly slid into public awareness over the past decade. With the rates of perceived stigma decreasing from 64 to 46 percent and personal stigma decreasing from 11 to 6 percent, it seems that there has been a collective effort to address this invisible issue that has been willfully ignored and demonized for the better part of history (Eisenberg & Lipson, 2019). According to WHO, mental health conditions and substance use disorders have risen by 13%, listing suicide as the second leading cause of death for people aged 15 to 29 ("Mental health", n.d.). While these statistics seem at odds with one another, it is important to keep in mind survivorship bias, that is, the logical error that concentrates on the successful, more visible party. In this case, this sharp surge of patients may be a positive result of mental health awareness and de-stigmatization as more individuals are willing to seek aid, rather than fall victim to the criticism of a "weak generation". These results, of course, are not without effort. Mental health campaigns, media representation, and open discussion have all facilitated this social transition. In a tandem campaign and study duo, CAMH concluded that their mass media campaign titled "Transforming Lives" prompted an increase in the number of psychiatric emergency visits ("Mental health awareness campaign leads to increase in the number of people seeking help, new CAMH study reveals", n.d.). Indeed, though the data shows a rise in clinical diagnoses, they are also correlated with increased treatment, with studies revealing a higher improvement rate with long term therapies (de Maat et al., 2009).

Defining Treatment Resistance

Modern therapy and pharmacology has taken great strides in improving the dispositions of individuals suffering from mood and psychotic disorders, and there seems to be a global social improvement in the state of mental health issues. With this in mind, this chapter now turns to defining treatment resistance in psychiatry, which is defined by the American Psychological Association as the "failure of a disease or illness to respond positively or significantly to treatment" ("APA Dictionary of Psychology", n.d.). This also includes a patient's non adhering behaviour or refusal to follow recommended medical and/ or psychological recovery plans. While the definition and number of failed treatments for a treatment resistance are not standardized, there is a general consensus of a requirement of exhausting a minimum of two ineffective trials, rendering them unable to work, attend school, or maintain healthy relationships (Brown et al., 2019). This label is not limited to a specific disease but is rather a designation that may include mood and anxiety, eating, obsessive-compulsive, personality, and substance related illnesses. This diverse range gives rise to different root causes and prevalence, the most common being mood disorders, such as depression. This chapter will broadly explore several of the most common treatment resistance disorders and why they may occur.

Treatment Resistance in Depression

Depression is perhaps one of the most well researched areas concerning treatment resistance. Classified as a mood disorder associated with feelings of sadness, loss, and apathy that persists over two weeks, it is an illness that affects more than 264 million people worldwide (James et al., 2018). With symptoms varying from mild, such as loss of energy and changes in sleep patterns, to the most severe being self harm and suicide, this is a condition brought on by biochemistry, genetics, medical conditions, and personality and environmental factors ("What Is Depression?", 2020). Biologically, depression occurs due to an imbalance of neurotransmitters which results in a lack of norepinephrine, serotonin, and dopamine in circulation. There are several options to attempt before resorting to a treatment resistant label. Standard initial care for mild to severe depression including antidepressant medications such as selective serotonin reuptake inhibitors (SSRIs) which target the neurotransmitters to inhibit reuptake of serotonin in the synapse

(Larsen et al., 2020). Depending on patient preference and drug specific factors, tricyclic antidepressants, mirtazapine, bupropion, and venlafaxine are other first line alternatives to SSRIs (Grover et al., 2017). Medical treatment has a 60 percent improvement rate alone, but psychotherapeutic interventions can also be used separately or concurrently to expedite recovery (Boseley, 2018). In particular, cognitive behavioural therapy (CBT) focuses on adjusting information processing while interpersonal psychotherapy focuses on changing interpersonal behavioural patterns that facilitate the illness in question (Stangier, 2011). Both approaches have the highest depression management success rate with CBT and interpersonal therapy seeing improvement in 64.7% and 75% in depressed adolescents respectively (Mufson, 1999). Psychotherapeutic substitutes such as supportive, behaviour, martial, family, and brief psychodynamic psychotherapy can be considered based on patient factors.

Treatment resistant depression occurs in 50% to 60% of cases (Fava, 2003). Antidepressants may be ineffective when doses are skipped due to nonadherence or when not given enough time to take effect. Even when correctly dosage and compliance, biochemical causes of mental illnesses vary and no one drug is sufficient for all. One individual's condition may be rooted in environmental or genetic factors rather than being a synaptic issue, rendering neurotransmitter targeted medication inadequate ("Why Antidepressants Don't Work For So Many", 2009). Genetics and health conditions may also play a role in the efficacy of medication, with heart disease, cancer, thyroid problems, and substance abuse being major contributors to depression and potential medicine incompatibilities (Causes of Treatment-Resistant Depression, 2020). In terms of therapy, a type of nonadherence resistance specific to depression involves the inability to accept. According to Dr. David Burns who popularized CBT, some patients may "cling to depression" and avoid prescribed regimes as a means to avoid processing internal flaws or outward conditions (Burns, 2017). While they may want to recover, they may utilise their diagnosis to bypass confronting the more prevalent issues in their lives and decide to not involve themselves with the necessary steps to rehabilitation.

Treatment Resistance in Schizophrenia

Schizophrenia is a chronic mental illness that, when active, may cause hallucinations, delusions, psychosis and disorganized thought and speech patterns ("What Is Schizophrenia?", n.d.). Common manifestations of the disorder include hearing voices, seeing things that are not there, or holding false beliefs. These symptoms can be classified into either positive or negative, where the positive include shifts in behaviour, thinking, and distortion of reality, while the negative presents itself as social withdrawal, lethargy, and apathy (Burton & Davison, 2012). With around 20 million diagnosed in the world, it is a comparative uncommon disease, leading to heightened stigma and misconception (James et al., 2018). While the media plays upon harmful stereotypes for the purpose of entertainment, most individuals with schizophrenia are no more dangerous or violent than the general public, nor do their illness cause "split personalities". The unfortunate fact of the matter is that patients suffering from schizophrenia are more likely to be a danger to themselves rather than others, with a rate of suicide that is 20 times higher than the population average (Zaheer et al., 2020). Potential explanations for the disorder include a combination of genetics, where heredity increases the likelihood of developing schizophrenia by six times (Chou et al., 2016). Similar to depression, pathophysiological research has found abnormalities in neurotransmission in the diagnosed (Patel et al., 2014). Most theories focus on an imbalance of dopamine, serotonin, and glutamate and irregular connections in the default mode network which links the different regions of the brain (Dryden-Edwards, 2017). Other reasonings include environmental conditions and substance abuse. Ingesting hallucinogens, amphetamines, and other psychotomimetic drugs in adolescence can induce psychosis experiences and trigger predisposed schizophrenia (Davis, 2017). Though the severity varies and symptoms often lessen with age, there is no known cure. However, through a pairing of pharmacological treatment in the form of antipsychotics and psychotherapies such as CBT, the disorder can be managed such that the patient can lead a relatively normal life.

By blocking the D2 receptor, most antipsychotic medications can reduce excess levels of dopamine that induce positive symptoms (Li et al., 2016). Unfortunately, among individuals with schizophrenia, treatment resistance occurs in up to 34 percent of cases (Potkin et al., 2020). The dopamine supersensitivity hypothesis (DSH) gives some insight into the source of some treatment resistance cases and why standard pharmacological treatment is ineffective (Chouinard et al., 1978). It is suspected that extended blockage of the dopamine D2 receptor may cause biochemistry development in the brain leading to symptoms that are unresponsive to the original dosage, thus triggering potential relapses in the event of drug withdrawal and requiring increased subsequent applications (Potkin et al., 2020). Other research finds biological differences in treatment responsive and treatment resistance schizophrenia, where TRS patients may have heightened glutamate levels in the anterior cingulate cortex, increased neuroinflammation, as well as lower serotonin and striatal dopamine synthesis capacity (Demjaha et al., 2014). In TRS, improvement is more significant when diagnosed in the beginning stages of the illness, which would allow for an early and more effective application of clozapine, the only approved antipsychotic for TRS. However, clozapine only has a 40 percent rate of improvement and alternatives are limited. Electroconvulsive therapy (ECT) has been shown to be a promising substitute, with a more than 40 percent success rate when accompanying the use of the medication, but more research is required for the use of ECT alone as a means of improvement (Sinclair et al., 2019).

Treatment Resistance in Substance Use Disorder

Substance use disorder is a new term introduced in the DSM-5 that incorporates the previous editions' definitions of substance abuse and substance dependence, and contains subtypes according to the specific substance (Diagnostic and Statistical Manual of Mental Disorders, 2013). The Syndrome Model of Addiction theorizes that it is a single illness that has multiple expressions, but in most cases, regardless of the drug, the disease is diagnosed with the same symptoms (Shaffer, 2017). Specifically, substance use disorder (SUB) affects behaviour and thought patterns, eliciting the uncontrollable use of a substance associated with negative consequences that affect daily functioning. This can involve social problems, impaired control skills, and evidence of tolerance and withdrawal problems. Notable substances include alcohol, stimulants, depressants, and other forms of illicit drugs, and tobacco. On a biological level, substances become addictive by taking over the reward centre of the brain, affecting the use of neurotransmitters, and ultimately causing it to release more dopamine than normal. It is the continuous rise in dopamine levels following the intake that becomes problematic, creating a pleasurable sensation motivating repeated action (Potenza, 2013). In particular, the basal ganglia is the part of the brain responsible for motivation and can adapt to repeated substance use, becoming desensitized and fixating solely on the drug for pleasure ("Drugs, Brains, and Behaviour: The Science of Addiction", 2020). Studies have found that genetics play a role in one's vulnerability to addiction and the likelihood of comorbidity (Ducci & Goldman, 2012). Medication may also be included in treatment, with most pharmacological solutions targeting the brain's neurotransmitter receptor sites, which can detoxify, lessen withdrawal symptoms and prevent relapse (Douaihy et al., 2013). Beyond that, treatment of SUD includes CBT and other outpatient behavioural therapy, as well as residential counseling, the latter entailing structured and intensive care that utilises a variety of therapeutic rehabilitation techniques.

It is imperative to understand that SUD involves a largely social economic aspect, where individuals of marginalized groups, elevated rates of adverse life events, and lower income are at an increased risk (Spooner & Hetherington, 2004). This is conducive to substance use disorder having among the highest rates of treatment resistance, with a relapse rate hovering between 40% to 60% ("Treatment and Recovery", 2018). This statistic can be explained by geographical accessibility barriers, financial problems, peer group influence, substance accessibility, stressful conditions, and family conflict (Kabisa et al., 2021). Treatment is a long process, one that requires continuous monitoring and adequate amounts of time in rehabilitation problems, which may be difficult to obtain given the socioeconomic conditions patients face. This makes the consideration for age, gender, income levels, social environment, cultural background, and ethnicity especially important when creating a recovery plan ("Principles of Effective Treatment", 2018). Therefore, in SUD cases of high relapse rate, this may be an overarching problem of mismatching treatment methods, where the unique individual conditions mediating the illness is not being addressed.

Non Disorder Specific Causes of Treatment Resistance

Beyond the disorder unique factors listed above, there also exists overarching explanations as to why certain mental illnesses are unresponsive to standard treatments. Misdiagnosis and overlooking underlying risk factors may mislead professionals. Unlike most fields of medicine, traditional psychiatry relies primarily on identifying conditions based on symptoms rather than examining the physical organ itself. Since many illnesses share similar manifestations, it is imperative to be able to exclude alternative reasoning for experienced effects (Morris, 2019). For example, biological issues such as problems with blood flow, inflammation, head trauma, or sleep pattern may replicate effects of a disease ("Treatment-Resistant Conditions", n.d.). Incorrect prescriptions in response to misdiagnosis can range from being ineffective in mild cases, to completely exacerbating the condition in severe examples.

Comorbidity is a secondary cause of treatment resistance and is the simultaneous presence of more than one condition. In the United States, comorbidity occurs in 11.8 percent of the adult population ("5 Surprising Mental Health Statistics", 2019). Co-occurring conditions can prevent accurate identification and adequate treatment. Substance abuse specifically can greatly worsen the consequences of mental illness. The relationship is two way, where certain conditions are more prone to drug use as a means to cope or satisfying thrill seeking tendencies (Lesser, 2021). Among youth, over 60 percent of adolescents in US substance use disorder rehabilitation programs have symptoms that meet the criteria for another condition (National Institute on Drug Abuse, 2020).

Realistic resistance, as opposed to unconscious resistance is defined as disagreeing with the therapist's approach, certain techniques employed in the session, and phrases used (Rennie, 1994). This may also take the form of withdrawing, refusing to take medication or following regime plans, disagreement, or missing sessions. Noncompliance may also arise through no fault of the individual, but rather as a result of the disorder itself distorting behaviour and thought patterns. For example, anosognosia is the condition where the patient lacks the ability to accept their diagnosis, and some cases of schizophrenia or bipolarism in particular may refuse treatment because they do not think they require it.

Lastly, beyond just the medicinal and therapeutic approach, it is important to resolve all issues that play a role in the illness. A support network is incredibly important in overseeing healing, where patients who lack family and friends face a more difficult recovery process. Accessibility to resources, economic conditions, and social groups can influence or trigger one's propensity towards treatment setbacks.

Conclusion

There are a multitude of different reasonings as to why treatment resistance occurs. While this chapter focused primarily upon depression, schizophrenia, and substance use disorder, unresponsiveness can also be found in select cases of bipolar, anxiety, and attention deficit disorders. In considering that these diseases are oftentimes chronic, the term "treatment resistance" may lend itself to be more on the insensitive side (Oaklander, 2017). It suggests that the end goal of treatment is the complete elimination of the illness when in reality, this is rarely achievable. Instead, it would be more accurate to commit to a path of recovery, for a patient to lead a fulfilling life despite the limitations of their condition (Demyttenaere, 2019). In realizing this, the author hopes one will take into consideration the many nuances and struggles of mental disorders highlighted in this chapter and ultimately develop a better understanding and empathy regarding the conversation surrounding mental health.

How Prevalent is Treatment Resistance in our World?

by David Supina

The prevalence of treatment resistance in Psychiatry varies depending on what specifically is being treated. According to one source:

- Those with schizophrenia may not respond to a couple different medications at a rate of around 30%.

- For those with substance addictions, the relapse rate is somewhere between 40-60%.

- As many as a third of those with depression may not experience full relief from their symptoms after multiple courses of treatment.

- Around 40% of those with anxiety may not experience significant relief of their symptoms from treatment.

- While specific numbers are not cited for bipolar, it seems to at least be prevalent to be a concern.

- Up to 80% of those with ADHD do not persist with their treatment plan. (Amen Clinics, 2021)

Of course, with the difficulty there can be in sorting people into whether or not they count as treatment resistant, there is some fuzziness that may be intrinsic to the numbers. Let's dig a little bit more into some research for the categories listed above (ADHD, depression, anxiety, bipolar, substance use, schizophrenia).

Schizophrenia

While the definition of what is meant by the term "Treatment Resistance" is covered elsewhere in this book, it is certainly relevant here. We will endeavour only to explore the question, however, insofar as it affects our subject of the prevalence of Treatment Resistance. It does seem that it affects us here, as one study found that depending on the criteria used to define Treatment Resistance for those with schizophrenia, the label could apply to 11%, 13% or 44% of patients. And another study by the same author reported a rate of 17%.

Part of the problem is that "[t]he definition of treatment resistance is reported inconsistently across studies, and there is currently no International Statistical Classification of Diseases and Related Health Problems (ICD) code for TRS [treatment resistant schizophrenia], nor does Diagnostic and Statistical Manual of Mental Disorders (DSM)-5 include a diagnostic code." (Morup et al., 2020, p. 2) This may explain why there are going to be potentially variable numbers reported, even if they are confined to a specific field: how do you settle on a consensus number if you don't have a single definition of the criteria? However, with schizophrenia, it does seem that there is a sense that the data rate of 30% is a little high, with their own estimate coming in at approximately 22% of those with schizophrenia would also be considered treatment resistant. (Morup et al., 2020)

Substance Abuse

It's worth noting that the prevalence of treatment resistance can be profoundly affected by the attitude of the patient toward his or her treatment. This is seen in the case of substance abuse, where those who are being compelled to treatment can be youth who see no particular problems with their habits, and are compelled by parents or other authority figures to seek treatment.
(Orr-Brown, D.E. & Siebert, D.C., 2007)

While this may be clearest in the case of substance abuse, it's almost inconceivable that it couldn't be a factor in other areas of psychiatric treatment. While it need not necessarily look like an out-of-control youth who sees no problems with their drinking on drug use, could not a similar effect be seen if the patient is, say, despairing of the efficacy of any particular treatment? If a person is already depressed, how hard would it be to then say that "there is no hope of getting better"? Or if someone is already struggling with their inattention due to ADHD, what stops a person from saying to themselves "I will never remember to take my medication anyway, so why bother?" This is, however, mere speculation.

A similar effect may be seen among prisoners, who may be forced into treatment programs by a court order, rather than seeking help themselves. In three different groups, the rate of treatment resistance among prisoners who were there involuntarily was higher than those who had elected to be there. It's observed that "belief by participants, that they are in treatment voluntarily, can reduce treatment resistance by as much as 20%." (Shearer, 2002, p.42) Even taking into consideration that these statistics are for just an incarcerated population, the disparity between those who are willing participants and those who are coerced into treatment should result in a similar disparity of treatment resistance, even the percentages differ somewhat. (Shearer, 2002)

Substance Use in Treatment Resistant Depression

There is overlap between a substance use disorder and depression, as up to 40% of those with depression also have a substance use disorder at some portion of their life, with the most commonly abused substance being alcohol. The correlation between treatment resistance and a substance use disorder seems a little tentative, with one study finding no particular correlation, though the same study did find there was one if the patient was using alcohol and another drug, their outcomes were worse. However, the opposite relationship, where those who had treatment resistant depression were demonstrably more likely to experience substance use disorder, both among those who had a previously existing substance use disorder and those who had not. This link does seem to check out intuitively; if prescription medication and treatment don't result in the therapeutic effects that one might hope for, it might seem like the use and abuse of a drug may seem better than just wallowing in a depression that won't go away. And if one is already depressed, the rational decision making facilities could be compromised anyway. (Brenner et al, 2019)

121,669 patients with depression were surveyed, of which, 15,631, or approximately 13%, were considered to be treatment resistant, so the sample size for this particular study was fifteen thousand and change. There was noted to be a high correlation between those who were treatment resistant and substance use disorder if they also had a personality disorder, but given that the fraction of people who also had a personality disorder amongst those in the treatment resistant group was only about 3% of the fifteen or so thousand, they excluded those results. There did seem to be an elevated risk of treatment resistant depression in those who also had a substance use disorder, though the likelihood seemed higher for treatment resistance in those who had a substance use disorder for more than five years. Those who had a substance use disorder specifically in the area of alcohol were far less likely than those with other substance abuse disorders to experience treatment resistance. (Brenner et al, 2019)

Depression

Given a survey of a few different databases, those had about 3,566 patients with treatment resistance out of 36,902 patients with depression overall, for a rate of approximately 9.7%. The majority of those who were classified as having treatment resistant depression were women, across all databases surveyed (though not an overwhelming majority). Those who had treatment resistant depression, unsurprisingly, went through antidepressants and antipsychotics at a faster rate over the course of treatment than those who were not considered part of the treatment resistant group. There is some difficulty in identifying whether a particular person is treatment resistant, especially since the patient may not be taking their medications as recommended, and whether a treatment has been tried an adequate amount of time to determine the efficacy of it as a treatment. Of those that had depression treated with antidepressants, approximately 16% were categorized as having treatment resistance. (Cepeda, 2017)

Anxiety

Approximately 60% of those with anxiety are responsive to treatment, which leaves us a rather sizable group that do not respond adequately. Of course, anxiety is a fairly broad category, as it contains "Obsessive Compulsive Disorder, Panic Disorder, Social Phobia, and Generalized

Anxiety Disorder, [which] are the largest and the most prevalent group of psychiatric disorders." (Bystritsky, 2006, p.805) When you factor in all these different variations, the prevalence of some form of anxiety may touch as many as 28.8% of the general population, who may qualify for at least one anxiety disorder at some point in their life, which when you combine it with as many as 40% of those who experience some form of anxiety as not responding to treatment (the estimates can vary between 10-40%), it is possible that a rather sizeable portion of the general population may experience anxiety with no obvious relief from conventional treatment. The sheer prevalence of some form of anxiety in the general population, when combined with the prevalence of treatment resistance, is concerning, to put things mildly. (Bystritsky, 2006)

Anxiety disorders can be underestimated due to their commonplace nature, but it can be dangerous on multiple fronts. One, it often is comorbid with other conditions. Two, in its severe or treatment resistant forms, it can have similar negative outcomes to schizophrenia. And even in mild form, the result can often be disability or even death. When it comes to the efficacy of treatments, perhaps 30% of patients recover through conventional treatments, while another 30-40% show at least some notable improvement. This still leaves at least 30% of those with anxiety who unfortunately do not seem to have the needle moved much by treatment. (Bystritsky, 2006)

So, what might indicate that a particular person might be treatment resistant for anxiety? This might be "related to severity of illness, comorbidity and presence of personality disorders and noncompliance with the treatment." (Bystritsky, 2006, p.809) However, a key factor might be inadequate competency on the part of the professional administering treatment. It might also trickle down to patients, who might not have realistic expectations of the effects of treatment, or just know what to expect at all from a chosen treatment plan. It really does seem that there is no single silver bullet answer as to why someone might be experiencing treatment resistance, and there are certainly people who have none of the above indicators and still seem to be treatment resistant. (Bystritsky, 2006)

Bipolar

As many as half or more of those with bipolar can experience treatment resistance. There can be a number of factors, but some that predict difficulty include "higher baseline severity scores, presence of [major depressive episodes] in the previous year, poor social functioning predict failure to achieve remission or recovery in [bipolar]". (Fornaro et al., 2020, p.2) Additionally, prevalence of manic or hypo-manic states, or mixed states (a mix between depressed and manic states), or the number of days with an elevated mood may predict the prevalence of treatment resistant bipolar. In fact, the presence of mixed states was found to be highly predictive of treatment resistant bipolar overall, especially when the definition of a mixed state is taken a little more broadly. (Fornaro et al., 2020)

While this group consists of more than those that experience treatment resistance, as many as 90% of people with bipolar experience some kind of relapse. And even among those who respond, there can still be mild symptoms that persist through effective treatment. A variety of effects may affect the responsiveness of a person with bipolar to drug treatments, such as "such as gender, ethnicity, age, smoking, diet, psychiatric diagnosis, disease status and concomitant medications" (Casetta et al., 2019, p.288) as well as genetic factors. Those who display low compliance are often associated with worse outcomes, and compliance is often lower with those who have psychopathology, who tend to experience more adverse reactions to medication. (Casetta et al., 2019)

Attention Deficit Hyperactivity Disorder (ADHD)

It is difficult to ascertain treatment resistance specifically in ADHD, as it appears this may be an area that needs further study, there is some interesting data in how ADHD behaves when it is comorbid with depression, and also with a learning disorder, specific learning disorder (SLD).

There can be a significant factor of comorbidity between ADHD and treatment resistant depression. Of those that experienced treatment resistant depression, about 34% had previously undetected ADHD, as opposed to only 12.7% of those who had non-treatment resistant depression. This can manifest in lesser outcomes. It has been difficult to estimate the comorbidity of those with major depressive disorder and ADHD, but the estimates range from 22% to 74%, which, even with the most conservative estimate, seems higher than the prevalence of ADHD in the general population. It is possible the prevalence of their comorbidity has to do with the fact that both involve some dysregulation of dopamine and serotonin, two important chemicals in the brain. Anhedonia, which means a reduced ability to feel pleasure, is a feature of both major depressive disorder and ADHD, and a potential predictor of treatment resistant depression. Among those surveyed that had treatment resistant depression, 57.6% had persistent anhedonia. It seems there are numerous links between treatment resistant depression and ADHD. The hope, however, is that if ADHD and treatment resistant depression are comorbid, that taking steps to treat ADHD (which is often not diagnosed at the start of the treatment for depression) may improve the outcomes for treatment resistant depression as well. (Sternat, 2018)

There does seem to be reason to think that if ADHD is comorbid with another condition, even another learning disorder, can lead to treatment resistance. ADHD is estimated to affect 7–9% of children worldwide, although it is difficult to extract from this fact the rates of adult ADHD, since not everyone who has symptoms that lead to an ADHD diagnosis in childhood have persisting symptoms into adulthood. It seems that those who have ADHD and SLD (specific learning disorder) are less likely to respond to stimulant medications than those who have just ADHD. By a number of measures, those who were diagnosed with ADHD (inattentive type, in the case of this study) alone outperformed the therapeutic effects of intervention of those who underwent the same treatment, but had SLD and ADHD comorbid. The conclusion here is similar to the case of comorbid ADHD and treatment resistant depression—both conditions need to be treated in order to gain hoped for results. The fact that this principle shows up with treatment resistant depression and ADHD, and ADHD with SLD, seems to indicate the broader principle of the importance of identifying and treating all relevant psychiatric conditions, or a lot of difficulty might be found in achieving desired benchmarks of functioning. (Friedman, 2018)

Conclusion

While there can be different numbers reported depending on the study and the condition being considered, there does seem to be a fairly universal problem of treatment resistance in every area of psychiatry. There is still room for more work to be done, and toward that end a more standard definition of what does and does not count as treatment resistance would help, but there does seem to be a serious problem where a fairly significant percentage of the population does not, for one reason or another (and it may often have to do with comorbidity with other conditions), respond to treatment as readily as others with the condition do. This is a serious consideration for those who need to seek treatment, and should be sobering to us that even our best and most battle-hardened therapies, medicinal or otherwise, do not work for everyone, and it may take more work in order to get someone to recover than one might otherwise hope.

What Science is Involved in Treatment Resistance?

by Katerina Bavaro

Table 1: Acronyms used in this chapter

Acronym	What it stands for
fMRI	Functional magnetic resonance imaging
RPE	Reward Prediction Error
BOLD	Blood oxygen level dependent
HC	Healthy Control
TRS	Treatment resistant Schizophrenia
NTR	Non Treatment resistant
D2 Receptor	Dopamine Receptor D2
VAN	Ventral Attention Network
GSRD	European Group for the Study of Resistant Depression
GRIK4	Glutamate Ionotropic Receptor Kainate Type Subunit 4 (Protein coding gene)
CACNA1C Gene	Calcium Voltage Gated Channel Subunit Alpha1 C (Protein coding gene)
NMDA	N-methyl D- Aspartic acid/Aspartate (amino acid derivative)
AMPA	(a-amino-3-hydroxy-5-methyl-4-isoxazolepropionic acid), (mimics effects of glutamate)
MGluRs	Metabotropic glutamate receptor
BDNF	Brain derived neurotrophic factor

HPA Axis	Hypothalamic-pituitary-adrenal axis
spTMS	Single pulses of transcranial magnetic stimulation
MDD	Major Depressive Disorder
TRD	Treatment resistant depression
EGG	Electroencephalogram
GAD	Generalized Anxiety Disorder
NAA	N-acetylaspartate
GAD	Generalized Anxiety Disorder
SSRI	Selective Serotonin Reuptake Inhibitor
SNIS	Serotonin and Norepinephrine reuptake inhibitors

What Science is Involved in Studying Treatment resistance?

Functional magnetic resonance imaging (fMRI) plays an important part in modern psychiatric research. The technique emerged in the early 1990s and has contributed to significant advancements over alternative methods of studying brain function (Whitten, 2012). For instance, in a study done of differential neural reward mechanisms in treatment responsive and treatment resistant schizophrenia, it was used to observe the brain regions which were densely innervated with dopamine neurons. These typically show activation reflective of an RPE (Reward Prediction error) response which shows that the blood oxygen level dependent (BOLD) signal reflects the information the area is receiving and processing (Vanes et al., 2018)

For this particular study, the fMRI procedure was described as the following: participants were being tested for their response to a reward learning task which consisted in them choosing between two faces presented to them at the same time. This took place over a series of repetitive trials, for the purpose of them learning to identify which face had the association with a higher probability of receiving a reward (Vanes et al., 2018). This task was viewed by scientists as they observed through a head mounted-mirror inside of the fMRI scanner (Vanes et al., 2018).

The data gathered suggested that the behavioural response of the reward learning task between patients who had treatment resistant and treatment responsive schizophrenia (or non-treatment resistant) were similar. However, different neural systems were working to elicit the response between the two (Vanes et al.,2018). This will be discussed in greater detail in a later section. It will go specifically into the neurobiology behind non-treatment resistant and treatment resistant patients for various mental disorders. These include Schizophrenia, PTSD, Depression, and Generalized Anxiety Disorder.

There are other techniques which can be combined with fMRIs in order to study treatment resistance. For instance, a study was done by Etkin et al., which will also be mentioned later in the chapter under the section "PTSD". They used spTMS (single pulse transcranial magnetic stimulation) and an EEG (Electroencephalogram) as a technique in combination with a standard fMRI. The purpose was to address the limitations of traditional neuroimaging, in which the relationship between identified abnormalities in network interactions in patients and affected components of neural signal flow mechanisms was unknown (Etkin et al., 2019).

The stimulation of several cortical regions with the spTMS and the EEG working at the same time, made it easier to see results. Specifically, results that are effects of stimulation on signal flow and relate that to differences of fMRI connectivity. Therefore, it is a more specific way of looking at neurophysiological mechanisms. spTMs could be thought of as a brain mapping tool for understanding the neural basis of a resting state fMRI network measures (Etkin et al., 2019) . EEGs could be thought of as the signal result of spTMS.

Why is Treatment Resistance hard to define as a concept?

Within the field of psychiatry, treatment resistance has been difficult to define as a concept. This is because the evidence for distinct psychopathological or neurobiological features of treatment resistant mental disorders have been limited in terms of specific categories

(Demyttenaere, 2019). For instance, in Depression, Anxiety Disorders, and Schizophrenia, a definition has been agreed upon. One way of categorizing treatment resistance would be "an inadequate response to at least two adequate (appropriate doses and lasting for at least six weeks) treatment episodes with different drugs (Demyttenaere, 2019).

However, in other disorders such as in eating and personality disorders, it has been poorly defined. The central issue is that what is considered to be an inadequate response varies based on the disorder and can be defined differently in a first step treatment (the early stages of treatment) compared to a treatment resistant patient (someone who has repeatedly been resistant to different forms of treatment.

A response can be deemed to be inadequate based on the absolute threshold of symptom severity or can be a percentage change from baseline (minimum or starting point for comparisons) in terms of symptom severity(Demyttenaere, 2019). In Major Depressive Disorder (MDD) and Generalized Anxiety Disorder (GAD) a 50% decrease in symptom severity would be considered an inadequate response (Demyttenaere, 2019).

What is also problematic is that the outcomes in trials with treatment resistant patients often provide different results depending on whether the two treatment episodes were both retrospective (happened in the past), or whether one was retrospective as the other prospective (looking to the future). This makes it difficult to obtain a relatively homogenous population of patients due to this confusing form of categorization (Demyttenaere, 2019).

In order to combat this, classification attempts are moving towards basing treatment resistance on the number of treatments, with different treatments getting different weights. As well as episode duration and symptom severity(Demyttenaere, 2019). This is a step in the right direction as previous classifications such as non-resistant or resistant versus staging and the levels of resistance have made it more difficult to interpret study results.

What Neurological mechanisms are involved in creating these Treatment Resistant Mental Disorders?

There have been several studies done that show the neurological mechanistic distinction between Treatment resistant and Non Treatment resistant patients with mental disorders. In this section, four types of disorders will be discussed in particular. These include Schizophrenia, PTSD, Depression, and Anxiety Disorders.

Schizophrenia

Schizophrenia is a mental disorder which has both positive and negative symptoms. Positive refers to the presence of symptoms, and negative refers to the absence of such. Some of the most well-known positive symptoms include hallucinations and delusions. These have been thought to be the result of abnormal dopamine levels hence the dopamine hypothesis which has been the frontrunner in terms of the neurobiology of positive symptoms in schizophrenia. Specifically, an increased subcortical (below the cerebral cortex) release of dopamine augments D2 receptor activation due to a disrupted cortical pathway through the nucleus accumbens (Brisch et al., 2014). Antipsychotics, which are the main form of medication for schizophrenia patients, help control the symptoms of the disorder by specifically targeting dopamine.

As mentioned at the beginning of the chapter, specifically in the section titled "What Science is Involved in Studying Treatment Resistance?", was the Vanes et al. study. To recap, differential neural reward mechanisms were studied in non-treatment resistant (NTR) and treatment resistant patients with schizophrenia (TRS). Behavioural response to these reward mechanisms was categorized by reinforcement learning tasks. These were implemented to address dopaminergic functioning as midbrain dopamine neurons in particular encode violations of expected reward outcomes (Vanes et al., 2018). These are also known as reward prediction error signals (RPE) which are related to neural activation and the differential impact of emotional bias on these reward signals were compared between groups (Vanes et al., 2018).

RPE signaling in the striatum, which is a subcortical structure in the forebrain which consists of the caudate, putamen, and the ventral striatum has been shown to be reduced in patients with schizophrenia due to elevated presynaptic dopamine levels (Vanes et al., 2018). The striatum is the core structure of interest ,however the prefrontal cortex, parietal cortex, thalamus, and cerebellum are also relevant (Vanes et al., 2018).

This particular study took the assumption that had been underlying schizophrenia research that it was based on a dopamine abnormality and combined it with recent research that suggests elevated striatal dopamine synthesis is specific to NTR and anterior cingulate glutamate levels are selectively increased in TRS (Vanes et al., 2018).

The results found were that patients with schizophrenia did show impaired reinforcement responses compared to the healthy controls (HC). All groups, including NTR, TRS, and HC showed an emotional bias towards happy faces as part of the experiment was to choose between two faces in order to engage a behavioural response. The pattern of RPE signaling was similar in HC and TRS groups however for NTR patients they showed a significant reduction of RPE related activation in striatal, thalamic precentral, parietal, and cerebellar regions (Vanes et al., 2018). Therefore, there was a greater disruption of dopaminergic function.

What is implied is that mechanisms dopamine driven mechanisms underlying reinforcement learning in response to reward are selectively disrupted in NTR patients (Vanes et al., 2018). For HC and TRS patients on the other hand, issues with reinforcement learning do not come from RPE signaling that is related to dopamine. Therefore, TRS patients may not respond to antipsychotic medication because it specifically targets dopamine as it assumes an abnormality which is not the root cause of symptoms for TRS patients.

Emotional bias, which was part of what was being tested, showed a difference that was significant between NTR and TRS. This was in terms of how the RPE signal was associated with RPE signal in the thalamus and caudate during loss processing. NTR patients had strong emotional bias which was associated with a reduction of the RPE signal. For TRS patients, this was associated with an increased RPE signal. This is associated with the symptom of delusion for the TRS group (Vanes et al., 2018).

The data collected from this study supports the idea that TRS could have dysfunction not in the subcortical dopamine system, but in the implementation of cognitive controls that interact with this system. Perhaps it could be glutamatergic mechanisms (Vanes et al., 2018). This counteracts previous findings that the TRS group had a positive relationship between emotional bias and RPE signal during negative feedback in the bilateral thalamus and caudate which has been previously linked with dopaminergic dysfunction (Vanes et al., 2018).

To conclude, TRS can be separated from NTR based on different neural mechanisms underlying reinforcement learning. The findings support the hypothesis that a successful response to antipsychotic action would be based on dopaminergic dysfunction which has RPE signaling that departs from the norm. For TRS, it can be characterized by an abnormality of a non-dopaminergic receptor such as a glutamatergic mechanism (Vanes et al., 2018).

PTSD

The specific neurobiology behind Post Traumatic Stress disorder (PTSD) is complex and involves a combination of neuroendocrine, neurochemical, and neuroanatomical changes. The most common form of treatment is psychotherapy however this does not work for all patients.

Amit Etkin of Stanford discovered that patients with PTSD who had trouble remembering a list of words also had different brain activation patterns within the ventral attention network (VAN) (Etkin, 2019). The significance of this is that the network has the function of refocusing attention towards salient (important) stimuli. These people also tended not to respond to the intervention of psychotherapy.

This study took the approach that was drawn on the premise that disruption in basic brain information processing functions which underlie cognition create the foundation which various aspects of PTSD come from (Etkin, 2019.) PTSD tends to be quite heterogeneous, meaning there is quite a bit of variation among patients. Individual differences in cognitive capacities are related to individual differences in connectivity of the frontoparietal, default-mode, dorsal attention, and ventral attention networks (Etkin, 2019).

Neuroimaging studies in PTSD patients have also shown that in resting state fMRI connectivity there are abnormalities in large-scale neural networks (Etkin, 2019. Cortical regions were stimulated using spTMs simultaneously while recording consequent brain activity with EEG in order to find out more about this discovery. For more, see the section at the beginning of the chapter titled "What Science is involved in studying treatment resistance".

Results concluded that a neurobehavioral phenotype with the domain of PTSD does exist and is characterized by impairments such as delayed recall of verbal memory such as remembering a list of words and the resting state fMRI connectivity on the VAN. This phenotype was found to be associated with poor treatment outcomes. Using the fMRI combined with the spTMS/EEG technique the authors were able to find the particular cause. Using the spTMS/EEG to examine neurostimulation induced neural signal flow there was a particular neurophysiological circuit response associated with the degree of within-VAN fMRI connectivity.

The poorer connectivity had to do with a more prolonged circuit perturbation to single spTMS pulses delivered to the right sided anterior prefrontal VAN region. As a result, it showed up as alpha-range below baseline desynchronization (Etkin, 2019). The late alpha- range below baseline has been reported with motor cortex stimulation and may reflect a locked aspect of the response to spTMS/ EEG response (Etkin, 2019). It could be sensitive to agonists of either ▯-aminobutyric acid type A (GABAA) or GABAB receptors (Etkin, 2019). The desynchronization increases by drugs that stimulate the receptors mentioned therefore in patients where this is the case which is those who have lower within-VAN connectivity it could be a larger inhibitory response to the stimulation of the VAN (Etkin, 2019).

Depression

The neurobiology of depression features alterations in the corticolimbic system; a combination of limbic and cortical structures which is made up of several brain regions (Wohleb et al., 2016). These include the prefrontal cortex, the pituitary gland, amygdala, brain stem, hypothalamus, cerebellum, nucleus and accumbens and the hippocampus. There are also other structures that are involved however there has not yet been a general consensus of whether they are officially part of the corticolimbic system or not.

The alterations which go in the neurobiology of depression are dichotomous. For instance, the the prefrontal cortex and hippocampus exhibit neuronal atrophy (loss of neurons) and synaptic dysfunction, whereas the nucleus accumbens and amygdala exhibit neuronal hypertrophy (increase of neurons) and increased synaptic activity (Wohleb et al. 2016).

In 1999, the GSRD implemented a staging method for treatment-resistant depression. The criteria developed was under the notion that if a patient was resistant to at minimum two consecutive adequate antidepressant trials independent from the class of antidepressants that include augmentation and combination medications administered, they were considered treatment-resistant (Caraci et al.,2018). Discussed in a previous section titled Why is Treatment Resistance hard to define as a concept?" There have been issues in the past with defining treatment resistance as a concept. This is because there is great variation depending on the type of mental disorder and even variation in between patients. Also, different stages using this method of categorization do correspond also to the number of failed antidepressant trials.

Features which have been found to have a significant association with the presence of treatment resistance in depression include comorbid anxiety disorders, comorbid personality disorder, suicide risk, depressive symptom severity and melancholic features (Caraci et al.,2018). Others are also more than one previous hospitalization due to MDD, recurrent depressive episodes, nonresponse to the first administered antidepressant, and age of onset less than or equal to 18 (Caraci et al.,2018).

There is some genetic disposition to treatment resistant depression as the statistic is that approximately 42% of the variance in antidepressant response contributes to genetics (Caraci et al. ,2018). Depression, historically, has been defined as a monoaminergic disorder referring to the idea that it is as a result and sustained by a deficit of monoamine neurotransmitters. The four major ones include serotonin, dopamine, and norepinephrine. However, this theory has since been revised to include glutamate as a key player, which is part of the amino acids, but can regulate depression through interaction with monoamines.

Therefore, genes of interest include those involved in monoaminergic and glutamatergic transmission as well as synaptic plasticity. Antidepressants such as N-methyl- D-Aspartate receptor antagonist ketamine would be an example of this targeting these specific neurotransmitters (Caraci et al.,2018). GRIK4 has been proposed as the candidate gene for TRD along with Protein phosphate 3 catalytic subunit gamma,brain-derived neurotrophic factor and CACNA1C among others (Caraci et al.,2018). These are suspected mainly because of their involvement with synaptic plasticity mediated by a glutamatergic agent, which is derived from the glutamate neurotransmitter.

N-methyl- D-Aspartate receptor antagonist ketamine functions as an antidepressant. It does so as it involves two components, one being N-methyl-D-aspartate (NMDA) which has been found to play a major role in depression and the other being ketamine. Ketamine is a NMDA antagonist meaning its purpose is to inhibit NMDA actions. It also increases levels of glutamate which leads to structural neuronal changes. These include increased dendritic growth of neurons which can contribute to synaptogenesis and increase in (BDNF) brain-derived neurotrophic factor (Sattar et al., 2018). This can increase long-term potentiation and improve symptoms of depression.

GRIK4 as previously mentioned, has been proposed as one the candidate genes for TRD, it codes specifically for the kainic acid-type receptor KA1 which responds to glutamate (Paddock et al., 2007). Specific markers have been found to contribute to non-response to SSRIs such as citalopram and other antidepressants.

Protein phosphate 3 catalytic subunit gamma is a specific protein coding gene. It has involvement in the process of bringing in glutamatergic mediated synaptic plasticity through the modulation of calcineurin, which is a neuron-enriched phosphatase that regulates synaptic plasticity and also antagonizes the effects of cAMP-activated protein kinase A (Fabbri et al., 2014). The balance between kinase/ phosphate is critical for the transition to long-term cellular responses in neurons (Fabbri et al., 2014). Recent evidence has supported the idea that Protein phosphate 3 catalytic subunit gamma may be a gene which may make people more susceptible to both affective and cognitive disorders. This is because altered calcineurin can induce depressive-like behaviours (Fabbri et al., 2014)

Lastly, CACNA1C is a gene that encodes for the alpha-1 subunit of the L-type voltage dependent calcium channels and is involved in the modulation of synaptic plasticity (Caraci et al.,2018). A study that was done looking at pleiotropic genes in psychiatry found that the GO:0006942 pathway which is associated with the CACNA1C gene is a useful predictor of TRD (Fabbri et al.,2018). The regulation of calcium currents through L-type calcium channels played a critical role for expression of neuroplasticity (Fabbri et al.,2018). The genes found in this pathway were linked to long-term potentiation, neural survival, and neurogenesis, but also to MDD and antidepressant efficacy (Fabbri et al.,2018)

The role of Glutamate in Depression

Glutamate can affect neuron activity by rapid actions exerted via ligand gated ion channels such as NMDA, AMPA, and kainate receptors. It can also slow down modulatory action exerted via the eight (mGluRs) G-Protein coupled metabotropic receptors (Caraci et al.,2018). It has been hypothesized that a dysregulated excitatory glutamatergic neurotransmission in specifically the ventral anterior (subgenial) cingulate cortex could result in a functional hypoactivity, meaning it would be less active (Caraci et al.,2018). This would impact specifically the ascending monoamine systems which contribute to the onset of affective and cognitive symptoms in MDD (Caraci et al.,2018).

For patients with TRD, an abnormal cycling of glutamate and GABA has been shown with increased amounts in the occipital lobe. and a decrease in the prefrontal regions. It has been suggested by blocking NMDA receptors which is what N-methyl- D-Aspartate receptor antagonist ketamine does as previously mentioned. If it blocks these receptors specifically on GABAergic interneurons , ketamine will cause a rapid increase in extracellular glutamate in the prefrontal cortex (Caraci et al.,2018).

The process has glutamate release spontaneously happening as a result, which will activate AMPA receptors which will cause the depolarization of postsynaptic neurons. What will then happen will be that L-type voltage gated calcium channels will activate. BDNF will be released from the vesicles (sacs) which activate rapamycin which plays a major role in synaptic plasticity which is impaired in the prefrontal cortex of patients with TRD (Caraci et al.,2018).

BDNF also known as Brain Derived neurotrophic factor is well known when it comes to synaptic plasticity and neurotrophic mechanisms in terms of depression. The expression of the neutrophil is reduced in several brain structures as well as at the peripheral level (all neuromuscular structures outside the skill and spinal cord) or depressed patients. It was even found that in chronically stressed rats that there were reduced BDNF levels (Caraci et al.,2018).

It has been reported that pretreatment BDNF levels are directly correlated with antidepressant responses, therefore the neurotrophin expression can essentially predict the response to antidepressants. However the effect of medication in TRD does not necessarily have to do with the modulation of peripheral BDNF levels (Caraci et al.,2018). Nevertheless, reduced BDNF gene expression has been found in TRD patients.

Anxiety Disorders

The neurobiology of both mood and anxiety disorders are a result in the disruption of the balance of activity in the emotional centers of the brain. Therefore similarly to depression, the limbic system is also involved. See the section on depression to learn more about the corticolimbic system which combines two different categories of structures.

The hippocampus is important as it has inhibitory control over the hypothalamic stress response system and plays a role in the negative feedback for the hypothalamic-pituitary-adrenal axis (HPA). Hippocampal volume and neurogenesis in this structure have been implicated in stress sensitivity and resiliency in relationship to mood and anxiety disorders (Martin et al.,2009). The amygdala, receives input from the hippocampus, thalamus and hypothalamus is responsible for fear and aggression and also plays a role in the memories associated with these emotions (Martin et al.,2009).There is also a neuroendocrine and neurotransmitter pathway component as increased activity in emotion processing brain regions in patients with an anxiety disorder could result from decreased inhibitory signaling by GABA or increased excitatory neurotransmission by glutamate (Martin et al.,2009).

The original five anxiety disorders were known to be Panic disorder, Generalized Anxiety Disorder (GAD), Social Anxiety Disorder, OCD, and PTSD. Though OCD and PTSD have now been removed from the group of anxiety disorders (Roy-Bryne, 2015). Most clinical trials of these disorders document response rates of 50%-60% and remission rates of between 25% and 35%. Treatment resistance anxiety patients include patients who relapse after remission and the rate is 10% at 20% at 5 years, and 30% at 10 years (Roy-Bryne,2015)

SRIs are currently the first-line pharmacotherapy for anxiety disorders. Benzodiazepines, tricyclic antidepressants, and monoamine oxidase inhibitors are also used. There are also new drugs that modify GABA-ergic, serotonergic, and glutamatergic receptor complexes and ones with anxiolytic properties (which also have a use of being a sedative). These include antipsychotics and anticonvulsants (Dilbaz et al,.2011).

There tends to be quite a bit of overlap between depression and anxiety therefore the explanations for the neurobiology are quite similar. Studies have been done on a genetic disposition and it has been found that variations in the gene GAD1 explained individual differences in people with (GAD) Generalized Anxiety Disorder (Dilbaz et al,.2011). Neuroimaging was done between GAD patients and HC, where it was found that GAD subjects had higher ratios of (NAA) N-acetylaspartate to creatine in the right dorsolateral prefrontal cortex (Matthew et al., 2004). This is suggested as a marker of neuronal viability meaning the ability of neurons to survive or function successfully. However, those who had GAD who had self-reported childhood abuse had a significantly lower N-acetylaspartate to creatine ratio in this region (Matthew et al., 2004). Individuals with GAD also had increased activation in the right ventrolateral prefrontal cortex when viewing angry faces (Dilabz et al.,2011). In other words, GAD patients had increased activity in areas associated with fear in the brain.

The literature lacks specific neurobiology which contributes to the explanation of why some patients with GAD may be treatment resistant especially since up to 30% of patients may be treatment resistant (Iliades, 2019). For now, the general consensus is that inadequate treatment, failure of patients to comply with treatment, and having a comorbid condition all contribute to (Iliades,2019). Front line treatments such as antidepressants like SSRI or SNIS, benzodiazepines, and also CBT sessions should be added (Iliades, 2019). For those who fail to respond to these front-line treatments, second line treatments should be administered such as diagnosing comorbidity, adding treatment for such comorbidity, adding a tricyclic antidepressant with an SSRI, and trying atypical antipsychotics (Iliades,2019). Future treatments that are non pharmacological could include deep brain stimulation, vagus nerve stimulation, stereotactic neurosurgery and transcranial magnetic stimulation (Iliades, 2019).

Conclusion

To conclude, this chapter covered several aspects of treatment resistance. This includes how it's studied, why the concept is so hard to define, and the neurobiology behind it. Four main mental disorders were focused on which were Schizophrenia, PTSD, Depression, and Anxiety disorders, this is by no means an exhaustive list of all of the mental disorders which have an element of treatment resistance but they are the most common.

The purpose of this chapter was to provide a general overview and to showcase certain studies addressing this issue in practice. A simplified version of the neurobiology and scientific components were explained for optimal understanding of the major concepts. There was also direction towards what research in this field may look like in the future. However, this will be addressed in more detail in a future chapter.

How Do Different Environments Affect the Creation of Treatment Resistance?

by Kendall Caperchione

Introduction

Treatment resistance is a complex topic within the medical field and perplexes doctors and scientists alike as there is not one solidified answer or solution to the issue. The issue of treatment resistance affects both physical and psychiatric conditions and disorders, and in terms of psychiatric disorders, resistance is a major component since each person's biological makeup reacts to medication differently. Treatment resistance, as defined in previous chapters, cannot be easily defined or confined to one definition, but to understand the concept better most medical professionals perceive treatment resistance to be when a medication that is meant to deal with a disorder does not work the way it is designed (Demyttenaere, 2019). A singular definition does not adequately work for what treatment resistance can be defined as, since different mental disorders require different medical treatments as well as varied methods depending on the individual. For example, disorders such as depression and anxiety, treatment resistance is defined by specific medicinal measurements (how they affect the person over a specific time period), eating disorders are the hardest to define as each individual person reacts to medications differently, and personality disorders are included in treatment resistance as patients often resist treatment altogether (Demyttenaere, 2019).

This section aims to identify and analyze the factors affecting treatment resistance in psychiatric disorders through examples relating to resistance in depression, anxiety, schizophrenia, and eating disorders.

First, different psychiatric disorders affect people in multiple ways as they have side effects, behaviours, and chemical variations that are distinct in each disorder. Resistance occurs in virtually any disease or disorder as each individual's body composition distorts and changes how medical treatments respond in the body. Medicine doses and their efficacy is the second environmental factor that alters how treatment resistance responds. Depending on the disorder and the medication prescribed, resistance can have a higher or lower probability of occurring. Finally, lifestyle factors and certain individual circumstances also alter the way the disorders listed above and how they promote or decrease the likelihood of resistance.

As explained, treatment resistance in psychiatric disorders is very prominent and has been a contributing factor to the challenges that the medical field faces today. In hopes of analyzing depression, anxiety, schizophrenia, and eating disorders, treatment resistance environmental factors play the most significant role in the occurrence of resistance in psychiatric treatment. Arguably one of the most crucial factors that affect resistance is the type of disorder and how it affects the person.

Psychiatric Disorders and their Ambiguity in Treatment Resistance

Psychiatric disorders vary in effects on patients and the types of medication used for certain disorders are specifically tailored to the particular disorder. The four unique disorders that treatment resistance affects are depression, anxiety, schizophrenia, and eating disorders as they are four disorders that millions of people deal with across the world and are significantly different on a case-by-case basis (ADAA, 2021).

More than 265 million people internationally deal with depression and are often dealing with depression in a way that others can not entirely relate to. Depression affects people unpredictably as many important factors including age, sex, medical history, and environment play roles in the types of effects experienced (ADAA, 2021). With multiple different types of depression such as Major Depressive Disorder (MDD), Persistent Depressive Disorder (PDD or Dysthymia), and Seasonal Affective Disorder (SAD), the percentage and ratio of people who are treatment-resistant are nearly one in every three people with depression (1:3) (Souery, Papakostas, & Trivedi, 2006). Through multiple studies, it has been shown that patients diagnosed with depression have high rates of non-responsive behaviour when being treated with average doses of antidepressant medication. Specifically, considering a controlled study done in the 1990s by Maurizio Fava and Katherine G Davidson, an experiment with patients suffering from depression revealed (after administration of antidepressants) that approximately 46% of patients who did not respond completely to the medication given, almost 19%-39% of those patients did not respond to the regular medication at all (Souery, Papakostas, & Trivedi, 2006). A study was done later in 2003 by Maurizio Fava, and it was discovered that closer to 50%-60% of people with treatment-resistant depression do not respond well or at all to prescribed medication, and it is often the case that antidepressant medication has to be altered or re-evaluated on a patient to patient basis (Fava, 2003).

Like that of depression, anxiety disorders are some of the most common psychiatric disorders today, accounting for approximately 18% of the world population and millions of people in both Canada and the United States (ADAA, 2021). Different disorders that are encapsulated by 'Anxiety' including Generalized Anxiety Disorder (GAD) or Social Anxiety Disorder (SAD), are included in the types of anxiety that patients and different people have resistant reactions towards. With anxiety disorders, people tend to live poorer lifestyles (which will be discussed later in the chapter), and with nearly 40% of patients studied responding not sufficient enough, anxiety is a disorder that also responds to treatment in an ambiguous way (Bystritsky, 2006). Anxiety is also influenced by multiple different factors including age, sex, external environmental factors, and biological factors, all of which influence and change the way patients react to average anxiety medication (Bystritsky, 2006). Despite the universality of anxiety, the disorder and its counterparts are still understudied and not understood to the point of desire by scientists and physicians, which is also primarily the causation of the differences in prescription medication used to treat patients with anxiety (Bystritsky, 2006).

Schizophrenia is another major disorder that affects millions of people worldwide. Schizophrenia is a disorder that is also affected by physical and external factors, however, it is noted that most people are found to develop the disorder between the adolescence stage and young adult stage (typically before 30 years of age) (NAMI, 1998). This disorder varies slightly as patients usually become diagnosed with the disorder after suffering a disconnect from reality multiple times over a long period of time (approximately 6 months), and have the correlative symptoms that prevent them from living normally and functioning normally (NAMI, 1998). Schizophrenia is also a disorder that people often develop treatment resistance towards. Through a series of tests, evaluations and experiments with different medications, people living with schizophrenia are usually able to find a medication that subdues their symptoms, however, there is still a large percentage (approximately 34%) of people living with schizophrenia that experience treatment resistance (Potkin, Kane, & Correll, 2020). Similar to other disorders, differentiating from a resistance to a specific method or medication and resistance to all methods and medication is important as the ambiguity of schizophrenia and the biological factors that influence treatment resistance are likely to impact the patient in life-altering ways (Potkin, Kane, Correll, 2020).

Eating disorders are another category of psychiatric disorders that affect the behavioural and emotional regularities of a person. Typically the symptoms that affect people with eating disorders include unusual eating patterns and behaviours that affect different physical, social, emotional and psychological functions of the person (APA, 2021). Millions of people are affected by eating disorders, even though the disorder accounts for only approximately 5% of the population and is mainly found in young people whose average age range is 13-35 years (APA, 2021). There are multiple different specified eating disorders such as binge-eating disorder (BED), anorexia and bulimia, all of which have difficult treatment consistency as eating disorders are paired with incredible difficulty surrounding treatment methods and high relapse rates (Aspen, Darcy, & Lock, 2014). Eating disorders consume a patient's life, and because of multiple different reasons for cognitive resistance or subconscious resistance, a patient can be very hard to work with when treatment options arise. Psychological factors such as ego-dystonic or ego-syntonic beliefs can play a major role regarding the treatment plan that would best suit the patient as well as the likelihood that the patient will resist the treatment (Aspen, Darcy, & Lock, 2014). This continues to prove difficult in the medical and psychiatric communities as patient treatment plans vary greatly and are constantly changing due to resistance from internal and external factors.

Medical Prescriptions and their Efficacy in Psychiatric Disorders

Medicine and treatment methods are some of the most important factors that influence treatment resistance for case by case variants. Continuing with the theme of four major psychiatric disorders, the hundreds of medications and alternative treatment methods available for patients to use or take present the opportunity for some to find a prescription drug or method that works for them, however, there are still plenty of people who are chronically treatment resistant and unable to respond positively to medical treatment.

Depression has one of the highest resistance rates compared to the four disorders examined in this chapter, creating prescribed medication and alternative methods that vary in success for people as what might work for one case might not be sufficient in the next. Different antidepressant medications can be categorized into sections; SSRIs (Selective serotonin uptake inhibitors), SNRIs (serotonin and norepinephrine reuptake inhibitors), and TCAs (tricyclic antidepressants) to name a few (Ogbru, 2018). Since medication is a probable option for situations where the case is severe enough, the type of drug, how much is administered, and when it is administered are crucial for the efficacy of the prescription. For example, switching strategies, combination strategies and add-on strategies are all different approaches that physicians will take when undergoing pharmacological methods with patients, and the idea of these is to use multiple different branded medications for resistant patients (Bennabi, Charpeaud, & Yrondi, 2019). Many physicians will attempt to use medications to treat average cases of depression or related disorders and will incorporate both medicinal and psychotherapeutic options in order to create the best possible treatment for the patient who has resisted past treatment (Bennabi, Charpeaud, & Yrondi, 2019). The type of medication, also known as the brand of the drug, is another significant factor when considering the efficacy of antidepressants. After hundreds of antidepressant trials done prior to 2018, the National Institute for Health Research based in the United Kingdom found that certain antidepressants such as "escitalopram", "paroxetine", and "sertraline" (among others) were the most effective drug when used on patients with modern to severe forms of depression, providing a lower turnover rate (when patients would stop taking the medication) than other drugs compared to placebos (NIHR, 2018).

Similar to other behavioural disorders, anxiety has a very high rate of occurrence as well as the occurrence of resistance when treatments are offered. Since there are multiple types of anxiety disorders and multiple ways to treat any one, it is often difficult for physicians to accurately hypothesize the 'correct' medication for a particular patient. Social Anxiety Disorder (SAD), General Anxiety Disorder (GAD) and Panic Disorder with/without Agoraphobia (PDA) are some of the most common types of anxiety branches and are often treated through hybrid methods (Bandelow, Michaelis, & Wedekind, 2017). Anxiety can be dealt with through a therapeutic method, pharmacotherapy method, or through a hybrid that includes both medication and psychiatric aid. One method or the other might not work for a single person on its own, but with the hybrid method, some people who experienced treatment resistance beforehand would possibly be able to use a method that works for them and allows them to lead semi-regular lives (Bandelow, Michaelis, & Wedekind, 2017). As previously mentioned, approximately 60% of people who have anxiety are responsive to treatment options, meaning nearly 40% of anxiety patients have not responded well to treatment options. This is a result of multiple environmental factors including the efficacy of the medication and therapy methods employed for certain patients (Bystritsky, 2006). For example, typical medications that are prescribed for anxiety include SSRIs (such as citalopram, escitalopram, and sertraline to name a few), together with psychotherapy can improve a person's symptoms with anxiety (WebMD, 2020). Although these methods might be the best ones available in the medical and psychiatric communities, this does not mean that patients are guaranteed treatment that will work, and oftentimes, patients find themselves with treatment resistance despite the use of these methods and medications.

Similar to depression and anxiety disorders, schizophrenia presents interesting challenges when discussing and debating treatment options, especially considering the medication and psychotherapy options available. Unfortunately, schizophrenia is a disorder that will most likely leave the patient with chronic treatment options, however, with a diverse team of professional help and methods for treatment that are patient-specific for the greatest possible outcome, a patient can control and handle their disorder (MayoClinic, 2020). After completing tests and evaluations, the physician's most probable route is to first attempt pharmaceuticals and antipsychotic medication. Through different dosage amounts, different types of antipsychotics, and different combinations of medications, physicians are able to detect what works or does not work, and further adjust a medication route for their patient (MayoClinic, 2020). For example, if a patient with schizophrenia has attempted and different medical trials of medication and psychotherapy options, physicians have found a new form of antipsychotic, clozapine, that has had significant efficacy rates when schizophrenic patients were unresponsive to other treatment options (Conley, Kelly, 2001). With different prescriptions comes different efficacies in terms of how the patient's biology reacts to the treatment. Similar to other disorders, schizophrenia medication varies in efficacy based on the patient's biological makeup and external factors, but also the factors at play that affect the medication such as size and time of the dosage.

Eating disorders and other similar psychiatric issues that people struggle with are oftentimes ambiguous and constantly changing depending on the physical make-up of the person with the issue. Since eating disorders are dealt with on a case-to-case basis, more so than the other disorders discussed in this chapter, there are multiple treatment paths that can be pursued including medications, psychotherapeutic options, and nutritional development amongst others (MayoClinic, 2017). With eating disorders being a different disorder type than the other three that have been discussed, physicians will normally take a different approach to treatment methods, using therapeutic methods first and later using medications if needed. This is primarily because medication alone will not be able to help an eating disorder, in turn creating an environment where treatment resistance would be prominent until it is later paired with therapeutic options or nutrition counselling (MayoClinic, 2017). Especially considering the psychological factors behind eating disorders and how ego-syntonic elements play a role in the occurrence of treatment resistance, some branches of eating disorders are easier to treat than others as the psychology behind them is different (Halmi, 2013).

Medication and psychotherapy options in the four disorders are some of the most prominent and widely used methods, despite the continuation of treatment resistance, as patients vary and their physical and psychological reactions to the methods differ. Medical factors play a small role in the overall environmental factors that create a space for treatment resistance to occur, and the final one to be discussed in this chapter is individual case circumstances.

Patients with Psychiatric Disorders and their Individual Lifestyles/Circumstances

Every person on the planet has a lifestyle and habits that they complete every day. Whether it be the schedule they stick to because of a job with set hours, or an unpredictable schedule because of a family that has multiple commitments, a person's life and individual circumstances play a major role in the factors that affect treatment resistance in psychiatric disorders. Lifestyle and individual circumstances can range, however, in terms of treatment resistance it is important to consider how the patient takes care of themselves including their eating and sleeping habits, their personal outlook on medication and treatment for psychiatric disorders, and their biological make-up (for why or why not a treatment would work).

Beginning with Depression and personal lifestyles, people who suffer from depression and similar disorders have difficult times leading what they would consider normal or regular lives. Some of the major areas of life that professionals recommend people with depression change or develop further are their exercise output, nutrition intake, and quality of sleep (Winchester Hospital, 2020). The idea of self remedied situations is ideal for many, however, this can lead to the occurrence of treatment resistance as if the disorder is strong enough, it can still prevent the patient from functioning to their fullest capacity (Winchester Hospital, 2020). It is possible that with the state of the three major physical factors of nutrition, sleep, and exercise, that depression can become amplified especially when considering or using prescription treatments (Lopresti, Hood, & Drummond, 2013).

Anxiety disorders constantly create negative experiences for people as it is an issue that causes the person to excessively worry about particular events or situations. Through a correlation between physical factors of a person's life such as eating, exercise, and sleep and whether or not someone suffers from anxiety, there is an understanding that the impact is a negative factor in someone's life. Medication and certain psychotherapeutic methods are not as efficient as they are supposed to be, and because of this (and depending on the person), the physician is able to take other methods into consideration. For example, if a patient is unresponsive to medication but has responded to some degree in therapeutic instances, other methods that could be explored are herbal preparations, behavioural psychotherapist, and nonpharmacological strategies such as Deep Brain Stimulation (DBS) (Bystritsky, 2006). Through different methods that are employed by the physician, the patient's ability to attempt to fight against treatment resistance becomes better, and patients are better able to be engaged and involved in the treatment process as they are the ones that understand themselves the best.

Schizophrenia, as previously mentioned, is a unique disorder that has had a significant portion of its cases that have become treatment-resistant, whether it be towards medication or psychotherapeutic means. Lifestyle plays an interesting role in the occurrence of treatment resistance in schizophrenic patients, as a study conducted in 2018 out of Pakistan presented a correlation between the use of marijuana and treatment resistance in schizophrenic patients. The study took a group of 264 people who had a history of schizophrenia, examined their medical records and history, and further evaluated the relationship between marijuana influence and treatment resistance to medication and psychiatric treatment (Arsalan, Iqbal, Tariq, Ayonrinde, Vincent & Ayub, 2019). Although the study was targeted to a specific group in the middle east, this study provides the basis for other research to be done within treatment resistance in schizophrenia and provides a factor that influences the specific disorder group as it impacts the treatment negatively through physical resistance (Arsalan, Iqbal, Tariq, Ayonrinde, Vincent & Ayub, 2019).

Finally, eating disorders and their lifestyle effects change the way people with the disorder (or something similar) function during their day-to-day operations. Eating disorders can become detrimental to someone's life as any of the encompassed disorders are conditions that alter and free the person's compulsions towards food and indulgences (Monte Nido, 2020). As treatment resistance is prominent in eating disorders, the likelihood of resistance occurring either through conscious or unconscious means is high. Controlling the intake of food for a person with an eating disorder can take time away from that person, and the unwillingness to attempt certain treatment methods (that sometimes, but not always, affects a person with an eating disorder) is a negative impact on one's routine as it can create a decline in other areas of their life (Monte Nido, 2020).

Conclusion

In closing, treatment resistance factors are affected heavily by the environment surrounding the issue and the specific patient. Environmental factors not only affect the occurrence of treatment resistance in psychiatry, but through the examination of each of the four disorders, we are further able to understand how the ambiguity of the disorder, the medical prescriptions for each treatment, and the lifestyle/individual circumstances that affects the occurrence and regularity of treatment resistance. Through this, physicians and scientists can further develop treatments and medications for psychiatric disorders that commonly face treatment resistance, and continue to provide those professionals with the ability to prescribe and treat those with psychiatric disorders in an efficient and sustainable way.

What Controversy and Opposing Viewpoints are There Surrounding Treatment Resistance?

by Razan Ahmed

Treatment-Resistant Depression

Treatment-Resistant Depression (TRD) addresses a wellspring of progressing clinical and nosological debate and disarray (Fornaro & Giosuè, 2010). While no univocal agreement on its definition and explicit connection with significant temperament problems has been reached to date, a continuously more noteworthy number of confirmations will in general propose an amendment of current clinical nosology. Clinical discussions identified with TRD allude not exclusively to its definition yet additionally to the manner in which this last is imagined: the "sufficiency" of a preliminary also the meaning of "non-reaction" appear to be misdirecting ideas (Fornaro & Giosuè, 2010).

Metabolic syndrome

The ADA and the European Association for the Study of Diabetes (EASD) as of late distributed a joint articulation scrutinizing the clinical worth of the metabolic syndrome. Their interests were as per the following: (1) the rules for the conclusion of metabolic condition are vague, and the reasoning for limits is poorly characterized; (2) the benefit of remembering DM for the meaning of metabolic disorder is sketchy; (3) the legitimacy of utilizing insulin obstruction as the binding together etiology is questionable; (4) there is no unmistakable reason for including/barring other CVD hazard factors; (5) the CVD hazard esteem changes and relies upon the particular danger factors present; (6) the CVD hazard related with the condition seems, by all accounts, to be no more prominent than the amount of its parts; (7) therapy of the condition is the same than the therapy of its segments; and (8) the clinical benefit of diagnosing the condition is hazy (Chopra, 2020). The creators of the ADA/EASD joint explanation recommend an examination plan to basically break down how the disorder is characterized and to decide its handiness in foreseeing CVD hazard far beyond that of the individual segments (Chopra, 2020).

The ADA/EASD articulation brought about the distribution of articles in the lay press, including USA TODAY, The New York Times, and The Washington Post. The National Heart, Lung, and Blood Institute and the American Heart Association keep on supporting the utilization of the term metabolic disorder to depict a substance that builds the danger of creating CVD and type 2 DM and its utilization as an auxiliary objective for lessening CVD occasions after the essential focuses of smoking end, bringing down LDL cholesterol levels, and circulatory strain control (Chopra, 2020). They concur that further exploration is expected to refine the most proper treatments for patients with the metabolic condition.

In a new explanation, the ACE repeated their unique opinion8 that the term insulin obstruction condition all the more obviously depicts the pathophysiology of this condition and that it is a significant driver of atherosclerosis and DM and may assume a part in messes as different as barrenness, harm, and irregularities of liver capacity (greasy liver). The ACE explicitly recognized insulin opposition disorder from type 2 DM and CVD in light of the fact that quite possibly the main objective was to distinguish people in danger before such outcomes happened (Chopra, 2020) . They trust it has been useful to perceive the bunching of variables that increment the danger of an individual being insulin safe as a condition. Moreover, they attest that the idea is clinically helpful and has driven doctors to look for related danger factors and related diseases. A few perceived specialists have additionally voiced their feelings with respect to the clinical utility of the process with utilization of the idea of the metabolic condition (Chopra, 2020).

In July 2006, a joint explanation from the ADA and the American Heart Association in regards to this new contention was distributed at the same time in Diabetes Care and Circulation. The affiliations expressed that they stay focused on CVD hazard factor acknowledgment and treatment (Chopra, 2020). The ADA favors evaluating and treating "cardiometabolic hazard." The joint assertion focuses on the significance of way of life change, including weight reduction and expanded actual work. Addressing the idea of metabolic disorder isn't new. In the 1998 report, the WHO noticed that people with focal weight, hypertension, and dyslipidemia, with or without hyperglycemia, present a significant grouping, analytic, and remedial test (Chopra, 2020). They required a reasonable portrayal of the fundamental segments of the disorder and information to help the general significance of every segment. They additionally noticed that globally recognized models for focal heftiness, insulin opposition, and hyperinsulinemia would be of help (Chopra, 2020). Shockingly, after 8 years, we have not sufficiently responded to these inquiries.

Spravato

Spravato is considered disputable by certain individuals for two fundamental reasons:it's produced using a medication called ketamine; it can cause serious results. The dynamic medication in Spravato is called esketamine, which is produced using ketamine (Slowiczek, 2019). Ketamine is endorsed by the Food and Drug Administration (FDA) for use as a sedative. Notwithstanding, it's additionally taken as a "party drug" that is alluded to as "Extraordinary K" and can be abused (Slowiczek, 2019).

It's critical to take note that Spravato and ketamine are not a similar medication. The two medications are just accessible with a remedy from a medical services supplier (Slowiczek, 2019). Nonetheless, Spravato is just given at affirmed medical care offices and can't be bought for use at home. With respect to the second worry about Spravato, it can cause genuine results, including sedation (lethargy, inconvenience thinking obviously, or powerlessness to drive or utilize large equipment) and separation (an "out-of-body" insight). Since Spravato has these genuine results, the FDA has put limitations on its utilization (Slowiczek, 2019). It must be given through a Risk Evaluation and Mitigation Strategy (REMS) at confirmed clinical offices. The REMS requires that in the wake of taking Spravato, you'll be checked by a medical care supplier for in any event two hours. During this time, they'll watch you for results. They'll likewise ensure it's safe for you to leave the office (Slowiczek, 2019).

Atopic Dermatitis

Atopic dermatitis (AD) is a persistent, backsliding, provocative skin illness with continually developing treatments and the executives. Commonness of AD is constantly expanding, with 15% to 20% of children and 1% to 3% of adults presently influenced around the world (Tilles et al., 2007). Treatment of this infection turns out to be more unpredictable while considering the generous weight of AD and the fundamental contentions encompassing AD hazard factors, accessible treatments, and explanations behind treatment disappointment (Tilles et al., 2007).

Different elements, for example, advancing remedial suggestions, supplemental medicines, patient inclinations and capacity to cling to treatment regimens, and expected antagonistic occasions of treatments, ought to be viewed as while treating AD. All the more explicitly, there is contention encompassing the results of TCIs and the jobs of dietary disposal, nutrient D, and food sensitivity testing in AD (Tilles et al., 2007). Right now, TCSs are first-line treatment and TCIs are second-line treatment for AD; these treatments might be related with an expanded danger of harm. In 2006, the FDA gave a discovery cautioning for harm, including lymphoma, with the utilization of the TCIs tacrolimus and pimecrolimus. Be that as it may, as per a 2015 meta-investigation, there was no critical expanded danger of lymphoma with openness to tacrolimus (OR, 1.04; P=.68). Interestingly, a recent report revealed a five-times expanded danger of lymphoma with the utilization of tacrolimus (P<.001) (Tilles et al., 2007).

This investigation, in any case, may have included a misclassification predisposition as the lymphoma analyzed while utilizing tacrolimus was cutaneous T-cell lymphoma, a typical differential conclusion of AD. Later correlations of tacrolimus versus TCS use in youngsters with AD recommend a potential expanded occurrence of lymphoma with tacrolimus contrasted and TCSs (95% CI amended IRR, 1.00-14.06) (Tilles et al., 2007). Limits to this companion study included not representing the expanded danger of lymphoma with expanded seriousness of AD, bringing about a potential jumbling factor, as patients with expanded seriousness are all the more habitually treated with TCIs. TCIs remain a major treatment alternative for AD as they show negligible fundamental assimilation and unfavorable occasions just as more noteworthy long haul improvement of infection flares contrasted and TCSs (Tilles et al., 2007).

TCSs stay a backbone treatment of AD. Albeit a powerful drug, TCSs are vulnerable to tachyphylaxis, the steady decrease in viability after progressive dosages of a prescription, which may bring about an untimely change to a substitute medicine. Notwithstanding, there is clashing proof on the advancement of tachyphylaxis. Despite the fact that downregulation of corticosteroid receptors in the skin can happen upon delayed treatment with TCSs, this may not be the justification for decreased adequacy in all patients (Tilles et al., 2007). In a 2013 deliberate survey, nonadherence to treatment and the leveling of restorative impact in the wake of accomplishing introductory maximal reaction were two proposed purposes behind the advancement of protection from TCSs and backslide of sickness. Two examinations containing 12 members each exhibited this hypothesis of nonadherence (Tilles et al., 2007). Patients with AD who recently bombed TCS treatment experienced improvement in EASI scores, pruritus VAS scores, and Total Lesion Severity Scale scores with desoximetasone 0.25% splash and every day call updates. These examinations reasoned that the evident diminished adequacy of TCSs was almost certain because of helpless treatment adherence than to diminished reaction to medicine. Potential issues identified with adherence ought to be considered prior to ceasing a treatment and ascribing an absence of viability to tachyphylaxis (Tilles et al., 2007).

Disappointment of proper treatment reaction may likewise be because of the intricacy of a patient's treatment routine, as proposed by illness rules, as opposed to the actual prescription. For instance, the use of wet-wraps, a tedious and frequently baffling cycle, is a successful treatment used in cases impervious to skin therapies (Tilles et al., 2007). Yet, an examination researching 50 kids with AD showed no distinction in mean SCORAD scores between bunches treated with TCSs in addition to wet-wraps or with TCSs alone (P=.445).Wet-wrap treatment is a troublesome method where people may battle in precisely applying the treatment, recommending nonadherence as a potential clarification for such findings. Additionally, when treating deteriorating AD, doctors regularly finish treatment rules using a reasonable methodology through basic rules like the Atopic Dermatitis Yardstick. However, this methodology expects legitimate utilization of medicines just as giving a full understanding to patients of the drugs in question, their strength, reason, and suitable dosing (Tilles et al., 2007). With such factor parts, it very well may be hard for patients to monitor their treatment regimens. It could be more valuable and compelling to consider easier treatment regimens as a way to improve patient adherence and accomplish wanted results. While assessing novel just as more seasoned treatments for AD, the intricacy of the administration methodology just as the patient's inclinations and capacity to stick to treatment ought to be mulled over (Tilles et al., 2007).

Bipolar Disorder

Regardless of the noteworthy expansion in prescriptions approved as successful in bipolar turmoil, treatment is as yet tormented by insufficient reaction in intense hyper or burdensome scenes or in long haul preventive upkeep therapy. Set up first-line medicines incorporate lithium, valproate and second-age antipsychotics (SGAs) in intense craziness, and lithium and valproate as upkeep therapies (Gitlin, 2006). As of late approved medicines incorporate broadened discharge carbamazepine for intense lunacy and lamotrigine, olanzapine and aripiprazole as upkeep therapies. For treatment-safe craziness and as upkeep medicines, various more current anticonvulsants, and one more seasoned one, phenytoin, have shown some guarantee as successful. Notwithstanding, not all anticonvulsants are viable and every specialist should be assessed separately. Joining various specialists is the most ordinarily utilized clinical methodology for treatment safe bipolar patients notwithstanding a general absence of information supporting its utilization, with the exception of intense craziness (for which lithium or valproate in addition to a SGA is ideal therapy). Different methodologies that might be compelling for treatment-safe patients incorporate high-portion thyroid increase, clozapine, calcium channel blockers and electroconvulsive treatment (ECT). Adjunctive psychotherapies show persuading viability utilizing a wide range of procedures, a large portion of which incorporate considerable thoughtfulness regarding training and improving adapting methodologies (Gitlin, 2006). As of late, bipolar misery has become a subject of genuine request with the predominant debate zeroing in on the spot of antidepressants in the treatment of bipolar discouragement. Other than state of mind stabilizers alone or the blend of mind-set stabilizers and antidepressants, a large portion of the methodologies for treatment-safe bipolar discouragement are generally like those utilized in unipolar despondency, with the conceivable exemption of a more conspicuous spot for SGAs, recommended either alone or in mix with antidepressants. Future work in the space needs to investigate the medicines normally utilized by clinicians with deficient exploration support, like mix treatment and the utilization of antidepressants as both intense and adjunctive upkeep therapies for bipolar turmoil (Gitlin, 2006).

Albeit most treatment proposals explicitly recommend utilizing antidepressants for intense burdensome scenes with the objective of ending them as quickly as time permits (with the expectation that the patient will keep on being on mind-set stabilizers), ongoing proof has recommended that more drawn out term disposition stabilizer/upper therapy might be useful for some bipolar patients (Gitlin, 2006). In two separate review examinations, bipolar patients who progressed forward antidepressants alongside their state of mind stabilizers had less burdensome backslides (32 versus 68% and 36 versus 70%) and no increment in hyper scenes. Moreover, in the bigger of the two examinations, patients progressed forward and supported antidepressants were fundamentally more averse to fostering a hyper scene. (P=0.003). Patients in these examinations were plainly a little subgroup of the all out bipolar discouraged patient populace. In any case, these review examinations recommend that some bipolar patients whose ailment is overwhelmed by miseries may do best on an upkeep mix of state of mind stabilizers and antidepressants (Gitlin, 2006).

Evolution of Treatment

The treatment of mental patients presents huge difficulties to the clinical local area, and a multidisciplinary way to deal with analysis and the executives is fundamental to work with ideal consideration. Specifically, the neurosurgical treatment of mental problems, or "psychosurgery," has held interest all through mankind's set of experiences as a possible technique for affecting conduct and awareness (Staudt et al., 2019). Early proof of such strategies can be followed to ancient times, and primes prospered in the nineteenth and mid 20th century with more noteworthy understanding into cerebral useful and anatomic restriction. In any case, any conversation of psychosurgery constantly conjures debate, as the boundless and aimless utilization of the transorbital lobotomy during the 20th century brought about significant moral consequences that continue right up until today. The simultaneous improvement of compelling psychopharmacological medicines for all intents and purposes killed the need and want for psychosurgical strategies, and in like manner the examination and practice of psychosurgery was torpid, however not neglected. There has been a new resurgence of interest for non-ablative treatments, due to some degree to current advances in useful and primary neuroimaging and neuromodulation innovation (Staudt et al., 2019). Specifically, profound mind incitement is a promising treatment worldview with the possibility to tweak unusual pathways and organizations involved in mental sickness states. Despite the fact that there is excitement in regards to these new progressions, it is critical to ponder the logical, social, and moral contemplations of this questionable field (Staudt et al., 2019).

The administration of mental problems is testing and frequently requires a multimodal way to deal with conclusion and treatment. There is a rich history of development in the field, driven by researchers, doctors and specialists. Specifically, the neurosurgical treatment of mental problems has a long and turbulent history full of discussion (Staudt et al., 2019). Nonetheless, the tradition of "psychosurgery" has likewise led to the improvement of current norms for examination and morals, and has encouraged a more profound comprehension of the pathophysiology of human conduct. Despite the fact that there is proof of psychosurgery traversing different millennia all through mankind's set of experiences, the most energizing, yet in addition provocative advancements have been inside the previous century, inferable from the consolidated endeavors of researchers and doctors (Staudt et al., 2019). During the 1950s, ablative medical procedures became undesirable because of the ascent of successful pharmacology and extraordinary expert and public analysis, in spite of the fact that exploration and practice proceeded with more thorough principles. Albeit the advanced therapy of mental problems is essentially clinical, the high rate of treatment obstruction and disappointment has encouraged a reestablished revenue in careful medicines with a non–ablative core interest (Staudt et al., 2019). In spite of a background marked by debate, interest in the capability of medical procedure for mental problems has persevered through and surprisingly expanded inside the previous few decades, fundamentally determined by the expansion and accomplishment of neuromodulation and by upgrades in primary and utilitarian neuroimaging. It is imperative to see improvements in psychosurgery with regards to the chronicled and ebb and flow comprehension of the neurobiology and pathophysiology of cognizance and conduct, the accessible therapies for mental problems, and the adherence to (or deficiency in that department) research morals (Staudt et al., 2019).

What Future Direction is Treatment Resistance Research Moving In?

by Megha Sharma

Patients with significant despondency react to stimulant treatment, however 10%–30% of them don't improve or show an incomplete reaction combined with utilitarian hindrance, low quality of life, self destruction ideation and endeavors, self-harmful conduct, and a high backslide rate (Al-Harbi, 2012). The point of this paper is to audit the helpful choices for treating safe significant burdensome problems, just as assessing further restorative alternatives. Treatment-safe misery, a complex clinical issue brought about by different danger factors, is focused by coordinated helpful methodologies, which incorporate improvement of prescriptions, a blend of antidepressants, exchanging of antidepressants, and increase with non-antidepressants, psychosocial and social treatments, and substantial treatments including electroconvulsive treatment, dull transcranial attractive incitement, attractive seizure treatment, profound mind incitement, transcranial direct flow incitement, and vagus nerve incitement.

As an end product, in excess of 33% of patients with treatment-safe sorrow will in general accomplish reduction and the rest keep on experiencing lingering manifestations (Al-Harbi, 2012). The last gathering of patients needs further examination to distinguish the best helpful modalities. More up to date biomarker-based antidepressants and different medications, along with non-drug methodologies, are not too far off to additional location the various complex issues of treatment-safe sadness (Al-Harbi, 2012). Treatment-safe gloom keeps on testing emotional well-being care suppliers, and further significant exploration including fresher medications is justified to improve the personal satisfaction of patients with the problem.

Major depression is a typical weakening problem influencing 10%–15% of the populace each year. Regardless of advances in the comprehension of the psychopharmacology and biomarkers of significant melancholy and the presentation of a few novel classes of antidepressants, just 60%–70% of patients with sadness react to upper treatment (Al-Harbi, 2012). Of the individuals who don't react, 10%–30% show treatment-safe manifestations combined with troubles in friendly and word related capacity, decay of actual wellbeing, self-destructive considerations, and expanded medical services use (Al-Harbi, 2012). Treatment-safe sorrow addresses an issue for medical care suppliers. Significant wretchedness with a poor or inadmissible reaction to two sufficient (ideal measurement and length) preliminaries of two distinct classes of antidepressants has been proposed as an operational meaning of treatment-safe depression (Al-Harbi, 2012) .It is accounted for that at any one time 14 million individuals experience the ill effects of discouragement, and just half of them get some type of treatment. Up to 70% of individuals who have sadness show significant improvement as estimated by usually utilized rating scales, for example, the Hamilton Rating Scale for Depression (HRSD),but they require extra psychosocial meditations for accomplishing total reduction. It is assessed that 10%–30% of patients with significant melancholy don't react to commonplace upper medications,7 and this gathering of patients needs preliminaries of an assortment of treatment methodologies (Al-Harbi, 2012). For this reason, it is especially essential to decide the sufficiency and result of earlier treatment preliminaries by utilizing the Antidepressant Treatment History Form that assists with barring "pseudo opposition" cases (Al-Harbi, 2012). Complete abatement is accomplished in 70%–90% of patients with wretchedness, leaving 10%–30% headstrong to treatment, and oversaw by an assortment of remedial modalities. Tragically, roughly 30% of patients with treatment-safe melancholy don't react to any treatment.According to the discoveries from the Sequenced Treatment Alternatives to Relieve Depression (STAR*D) study, half 66% of patients with discouragement don't recuperate completely on an upper medicine and 33% of patients do have an abatement of their burdensome side effects. Clearly utilization of an assortment of treatment approaches versus just an energizer makes the result variable in patients with significant sadness (Al-Harbi, 2012). Quite, the consequences of mega STAR*D contemplates open windows into the viability or inadequacy of energizer drugs among patients looking for treatment in genuine settings, remembering essential medical services, and assisting clinicians with settling on therapy choices in patients with therapy safe gloom . The commonness of both treatment-safe gloom and non-treatment-safe despondency would amazingly be variable across time ascribed to methodological issues, meaning of treatment-safe discouragement, and the remedial alternatives utilized, including neurostimulation therapies (Al-Harbi, 2012).Treatment-safe melancholy opposes genuine definition, however emotional well-being specialists concur that it ought to just be analyzed in patients who have not been helped by at least two upper treatment preliminaries of satisfactory portion and term. To add trouble to the meaning of treatment-safe sadness, treatment reaction and achievement has various implications across different exploration settings. Overall, treatment-safe discouragement dodges widespread definition and importance, and represents various demonstrative and helpful difficulties to psychological well-being specialists (Al-Harbi, 2012). The point of this paper is to survey the restorative alternatives for treating safe significant burdensome problems, just as assessing further helpful mediations.

There are five fundamental systems used to defeat a halfway reaction or absence of reaction to energizer treatment, ie, enhancement, exchanging, mix, expansion, and substantial treatments. Since there is no standard treatment approach, psychological wellness specialists offer the aforementioned techniques dependent on re-assessment of patients with treatment-safe sadness. The patient with despondency not reacting to energizer monotherapy requires an exceptionally individualized treatment plan and, as needs be, a few groups will react to a particular treatment, while others don't (Al-Harbi, 2012). Tracking down the correct way to deal with treat gloom can require a ton of exertion and time. Along these lines, the accompanying standards should be followed to oversee patients with therapy safe sadness: guarantee precise analysis, including subtype of sorrow; survey comorbid mental and ailments; assess psychosocial stressors, just as friendly and family support; guarantee satisfactory portion and length of treatment; screen and treat unfavorable occasions; teach the patient in regards to misery and antidepressants; guarantee consistency; and focus on abatement (Al-Harbi, 2012). The five methodologies are currently depicted momentarily.

Optimization of Antidepressants

The two center highlights of this methodology are to streamline dose and length of stimulant treatment for patients who have encountered just incomplete improvement. The upsides of this technique are to exploit the characteristic history of long winded despondency which dispatches over the long run and to balance the propensity of certain patients to cease the energizer rashly. Besides, it assists with recognizing a genuine suffering energizer reaction from a more transient fake treatment reaction. In particular, fake treatment responders have a more prominent probability of backslide between weeks 6 and 12 than patients who have reacted to dynamic antidepressants (Al-Harbi, 2012).An satisfactory preliminary of upper treatment has been characterized by certain clinicians as at least 6 weeks.7 If the patient shows a fractional reaction during this underlying period, another 4 a month and a half of treatment ought to be added. In this manner, a sum of 10–12 weeks might be needed now and again to get a full reaction to stimulant therapy.47 Irrational recommending of energizer prescriptions concerning measurements and length is a typical reason for treatment disappointment, and is basic in clinical practice. In an examination directed in an oversaw care climate, just 11% of patients requiring upper treatment got either a sufficient measurement or term of treatment (Al-Harbi, 2012). This nonsensical endorsing pattern is especially regular in old patients,and is particularly risky in low-pay and center pay nations (Al-Harbi, 2012). The more established writing recommends that normal remedy of maximal portions of TCA, monoamine oxidase inhibitors, and second-age antidepressants is related with a more prominent probability of reaction than more unobtrusive dosages in patients with treatment-safe depression.9 Notably, organization of higher portions of first-age and second-age antidepressants in quite a while with treatment-safe despondency requires checking of blood levels to follow the clinical reaction and to keep away from unfavorable impacts.

Switching strategies

The exchanging approach predominantly includes ending an insufficient stimulant and beginning another upper from a comparative or distinctive class in patients with treatment-safe sadness. Prior investigations discovered reaction paces of just 10%–30% for TCA in patients with a previous history of absence of reaction to TCA. A preliminary course of nortriptyline guided by plasma levels likewise proposed a 30% reaction in patients with an earlier history of TCA failure (Al-Harbi, 2012).Conversely, better reaction paces of up to 70% have been accounted for when patients are changed to an elective class of energizer, including the second-age heterocyclic antidepressants and SSRI/SNRI combined with an alternate system of action.Thase and Rush evaluated the applicable writing on old pattern exchanging approaches including a few inside and across classes of antidepressants in the populace with treatment-safe discouragement and comparative ends were drawn, with the suggestion to direct bigger, controlled, twofold visually impaired, hybrid investigations of SSRI/SNRI-safe despondency utilizing fresher antidepressants and TCA (Al-Harbi, 2012). Various generally all around planned investigations, which zeroed in on changing methodologies from SSRI in significant melancholy, have been directed to address these issues, and are summed up in.A rundown of the discoveries of these examinations is as per the following: reaction rate 26%–76%; reduction rate 28%–87%; a TCA may end up being a system of best option for patients who don't react to a SSRI; prejudice to one SSRI doesn't really mean bigotry to the entire class of SSRI; challenges incorporate gathering controlled information to address the similarly significant inquiry concerning the adequacy of an other SSRI when another individual from this class isn't powerful; across-class switch is a decent treatment choice; in patients inert to SSRI, organization of antidepressants with various components of activity is a compelling exchanging technique; and changing from a SSRI to a TCA and the other way around in patients who don't react to a 4-week preliminary isn't related with an improved reaction. The last perception contradicts that anticipated by current rules (Al-Harbi, 2012). The upsides of this methodology are improved adherence, decreased medicine costs, and less medication associations, while the disservices are that restorative increases from unique stimulant are lost, the patient needs to trust that the new specialist will get successful, and backslide or withdrawal manifestations along with unfriendly impacts may happen during the interceding time frame (Al-Harbi, 2012). This is especially evident if the half-existence of the main specialist is very long, similar to the case with fluoxetine (35 days), and another SSRI is begun before a satisfactory waste of time period has happened. Different antidepressants that require longer waste of time times of as long as 14 days are clomipramine, tranylcypromine, moclobemide, bupropion, and phenelzine whenever changed to another TCA, monoamine oxidase inhibitor, or SSRI (Al-Harbi, 2012). Serotonin disorder, reflecting harmful serotonin levels in the focal sensory system and described by hyperalertness, disturbance, disarray, anxiety, myoclonus, hyperreflexia, diaphoresis, shuddering, quake, and, perhaps, passing, may at times create if the waste of time period was deficient when changing starting with one SSRI upper then onto the next (Al-Harbi, 2012). In rundown, the dangers of harmfulness are more noteworthy with higher measurement regimens and a deficient waste of time period, albeit pressing cases may require a more limited exchanging span.

Combination of antidepressants

Combination treatment includes the option of a second stimulant specialist from an alternate class to the helpful routine of patients with treatment-safe depression (Al-Harbi, 2012).The extra upper is utilized for 12 weeks or even a very long time in ideal doses. Older antidepressants might be utilized on the grounds that they are accounted for to have great outcomes in treatment-safe discouragement combined with extreme, repetitive wretchedness. Different kinds of blend are accounted for in the writing, however the most well-known are TCA + SSRI followed by, eg, venlafaxine + TCA, SSRI + SSRI, and SSRI + venlafaxine (Al-Harbi, 2012). Venlafaxine + mirtazapine is oftentimes utilized in clinical practice, and this blend delivers a decent reaction in patients with hard-to-treat misery, which is ascribed to the synergistic activity of this mix. In one investigation of 32 patients with persevering burdensome disease, the mirtazapine + venlafaxine mix was given sooner or later over a 3-year time span somewhere in the range of 2002 and 2005. Clinical reaction rates were 44% at about a month and half at about two months (Al-Harbi, 2012). At half year audit, 56% of the first associate and 75% of those actually accepting treatment had shown a critical reaction. Altogether, 44% encountered some unfriendly impacts. Five patients stopped treatment because of sedation (19%) and weight acquired (19%).In another examination, the venlafaxine + mirtazapine blend was given to 22 patients with significant sadness who had bombed one preliminary of stimulant treatment. The mean length of treatment was roughly two months, delivering a reaction pace of 81.8% and a reduction pace of 27.3%. Just a single patient couldn't endure the mix, albeit half had critical results during treatment.This approach has certain detriments, ie, it doesn't take into account sufficient assessment of monotherapy, is related with decreased consistence, has an improved probability of antagonistic impacts, is inclined to polypharmacy, and has the potential for expanded medication connections (Al-Harbi, 2012). Benefits of the mix approach are that it is combined with a quick reaction, no titration is essential, introductory enhancements are kept up, the system expands on helpful increases, expansion of the subsequent compound is for the most part very much endured, and the weaknesses of exchanging methodologies are stayed away from. Also, the reaction rate is similar or better than drug replacement (Al-Harbi, 2012). In this technique, there may be a synergistic remedial impact, yet results because of medication drug collaborations additionally will in general arise, so cautious medication reconnaissance is required.

Augmentation Strategies

Augment therapy includes adding a subsequent specialist (however one that isn't regularly viewed as an energizer) to the remedial routine when there is just a halfway reaction to the essential upper specialist. The announced strength of suggestion for increase or exchanging is best supporting evidence.Various enlarging specialists, including lithium, abnormal antipsychotics, thyroid chemical, pindolol, buspirone, dopamine agonists, sex steroids, glucocorticoid-explicit specialists, home grown items, and more current anticonvulsants, have been utilized in patients with treatment-safe sadness (Al-Harbi, 2012). Increase choices, systems, and dosing techniques for the different specialists are summed up in. The central issues are as per the following: downregulation of focal beta-adrenergic receptors, which clarifies the 4–6-week delay in acquiring clinical improvement; lithium upgrades serotonin neurotransmission as well as effects other synapse frameworks and neuromodulators, with a reaction pace of 30%–65% in patients with treatment-safe melancholy who have bombed a few classes of antidepressants and combined with equivalent expansion adequacy at serum blood levels of 0.4 and 0.8 mEq/L; reaction may require only 2 days or up to 3 a month and a half, which is impressively more limited than the deferral expected with exchanging, which includes tighten of the principal medication, waste of time, and postponement in beginning of the subsequent medication; enmity of 5HT2A receptors, regular among abnormal antipsychotics, is likewise seen with mirtazapine and nefazodone and is combined with upgraded arrival of front facing dopamine and norepinephrine, which is believed to be a vital activity of upper specialists; fluoxetine-olanzapine revealed 40% improvement among patients with treatment-safe misery as contrasted and 30% and 25% improvement with fluoxetine and olanzapine alone, individually; olanzapine, aripiprazole, quetiapine, and ziprasidone had blended outcomes in a populace in with treatment-safe sorrow; T3 25–50 μg/day for 2–3 weeks is more compelling than T4 for expanding TCA, monoamine oxidase inhibitors, SSRI, and lithium in patients with treatment-safe sadness; checking thyroid capacity before T3 organization for a standard perusing just as after organization is significant; pindolol, a 5-HT1A postsynaptic enemy, speeds up the beginning of activity of antidepressants by forestalling negative criticism to the presynaptic 5-HT1A receptor however is presently not suggested for this reason; not at all like open-mark contemplates, buspirone is ineffectual in randomized controlled preliminaries; energizers had no certain outcomes in randomized controlled preliminaries including patients with treatment-safe gloom; in the wake of adapting to the choice inclination inborn in the STAR*D correlation of increase as opposed to exchanging, clinically significant contrasts in the unfriendly occasion profiles between these procedures were not noticed; risperidone (reduction rate [RR] 26.7%), valproate (RR 48.7%), buspirone (RR 32.6%), trazodone (RR 42.6%), and thyroid chemical (RR 37.5%) added to paroxetine 20 mg/day was successful and very much endured in 225 Chinese patients with stage II treatment-safe despondency; an extra multicenter preliminary of 183 patients with treatment-safe discouragement neglected to recognize a genuinely huge distinction among lamotrigine and fake treatment allowed for 10 weeks, yet post hoc examination recommended that future investigations of the viability of lamotrigine should zero in on explicit subgroups with wretchedness; a twofold visually impaired, fake treatment controlled investigation found that topiramate increase potentiates the adequacy of SSRI (fluoxetine, citalopram, sertraline) in the treatment of safe misery; and further enormous, similar, twofold visually impaired, randomized clinical preliminaries of expansion specialists in patients with treatment-safe melancholy are required (Al-Harbi, 2012).

Comorbidity

Patients with treatment-resistant depression should be evaluated for comorbid clinical and other mental conditions. This is obligatory on the grounds that 75.5% and 46.9% of patients with unipolar and bipolar treatment-safe gloom (n = 49) were accounted for to have at any rate one other Axis I and two extra Axis I analyze, individually, which included uneasiness issue and substance misuse (Al-Harbi, 2012). Hub I comorbidity has all the earmarks of being differentially connected with treatment opposition in unipolar and bipolar sorrow. It is likewise obvious with treatment-safe despondency, which is presumably connected with an assortment of actual infections at an etiological level, including agonizing disorder. Likewise, both physical and mental comorbid conditions add to treatment opposition in patients with sorrow (Al-Harbi, 2012). Patients with comorbidities who showed a fractional reaction to TCA, monoamine oxidase inhibitors, SSRI, and SNRI may get advantage from the utilization of energizers, ie, methylphenidate 10 mg multiple times day by day, dextroamphetamine 5 mg multiple times every day, or modafinil 100–200 mg once day by day. These meds are accounted for to speed up the impacts of energizer treatment, however have a potential for misuse and randomized controlled preliminaries neglected to create any treatment benefits. However, these meds may have a job in the adjunctive treatment of apathy.Nefazodone, another compound utilized simultaneously with endorsed meds in patients with treatment-safe sadness (n = 20) and high mental comorbidity (post-horrible pressure problem, substance use issue, and behavioral condition) delivered great outcomes, with half of patients (n = 11) showing considerable improvement, and a more modest extent having a more unobtrusive clinical reaction. Duloxetine and venlafaxine have likewise been utilized in a few examinations with genuinely great results (Al-Harbi, 2012).The essential standards of treating treatment-safe misery with comorbidities continue as before and all alternatives should be utilized successively.

Electroconvulsive Therapy

ECT is a perceived method of treatment for an assortment of mental problems, including treatment-safe depression.ECT is as yet the most reliably successful in patients with treatment-safe gloom, with a reaction pace of half 70%.Furthermore, ECT stays the treatment of best option for the most extreme, crippling types of treatment-safe wretchedness, however the strength of the suggestion of ECT is level C. Shockingly, backslide rates are fundamentally higher in patients with treatment-safe gloom after an effective course of treatment. Exploration is expected to set up the viability of elective techniques to forestall backslide following effective ECT, including upkeep ECT and blend pharmacotherapy methodologies. Patients who neglect to react to ECT as proposed in Stage 5 treatment-safe gloom address probably the most difficult cases. Indicators of nonresponse to ECT should be set up (Al-Harbi, 2012). In a huge patient populace with treatment-safe wretchedness, ECT was a compelling treatment for around 66% of cases. An absence of reaction to ECT was related with bipolar subtype, presence of hyper indications during sadness, somewhat less serious burdensome symptomatology, and extended length of the burdensome scene. In a new investigation of youths with treatment-safe discouragement, continuation ECT and support ECT were valuable and safe treatment methodologies for chose young people with extreme treatment-safe sadness, and manifestation reduction was accomplished without intellectual hindrance.

Future Treatment Options

New medications supported for the administration of gloom are available. These meds incorporate desvenlafaxine (a SNRI), escitalopram (a SSRI), and a reformulation of trazodone (Oleptro™). Various medications, including riluzole, that follow up on glutamate receptors and have upper movement have additionally been created and are supported for overseeing significant depression.Studies have investigated the part of ketamine, a NMDA adversary, in treating treatment-safe melancholy and intense self-destructive ideation. Ketamine seems to have a quick upper impact, inside the space of hours or a day, albeit these impacts just keep going for 7–10 days (Al-Harbi, 2012). Patients should be admitted to a medical clinic to get ketamine intravenously from an anesthesiologist, while their crucial signs are firmly checked. Ketamine is a medication of misuse and initiates daze like or dreamlike states. Like different sedatives, ketamine likewise creates gentle to direct intellectual results. Ketamine treatment might be likened to ECT and considering ketamine may uncover systems fundamental gloom and help to recognize drugs that can be recommended as antidepressants to a more extensive patient populace. In a relative investigation of 17 patients with treatment-safe despondency non-receptive to ECT and 23 patients with treatment-safe discouragement who had not recently gotten ECT were given a solitary open-name implantation of ketamine 0.5 mg/kg and assessed utilizing the Montgomery-Åsberg Depression Rating Scale at standard (an hour prior to the mixture), just as at 40, 80, 120, and 230 minutes after imbuement. Burdensome indications were essentially improved in the ECT-safe gathering at 230 minutes, with a moderate impact size (Al-Harbi, 2012). At 230 minutes, the gathering not presented to ECT showed critical improvement with a huge impact size. Ketamine seems to improve burdensome indications in patients with significant melancholy who had already not reacted to ECT. These fundamental outcomes warrant further examination in a bigger example size to decide the adequacy of ketamine in patients with despondency not receptive to other treatments. In one investigation, 10 members with treatment-safe melancholy were given riluzole, another NMDA enemy, alongside their normal energizer (Al-Harbi, 2012). Following 6–12 weeks, they encountered a very nearly 10-point drop on the HRSD.

In synopsis, 70% of patients with significant despondency react to starting energizer treatment, leaving 30% of patients who are recalcitrant to treatment and hence need exceptional treatment-safe gloom the executives procedures. 25% of patients with treatment-safe gloom will in general react to advancement and joined treatment standards and another half of patients are accounted for to react to exchanging helpful choices (Al-Harbi, 2012). Expansion methodologies focus on the leftover 25% of patients experiencing treatment-safe discouragement, with conflicting results (Al-Harbi, 2012). In general, in spite of the fact that there is no exacting compartmentalization of treatment reaction and reduction rate in the populace with treatment-safe wretchedness, around 33% of patients with the issue keep on being impervious to accessible restorative choices, and subsequently represent a significant helpful test to emotional well-being specialists.

.

References

Chatper 1 References

Beck, J. (2014, January 23). Diagnosing mental illness in Ancient Greece and Rome. The Atlantic.https://www.theatlantic.com/health/archive/2014/01/diagnosing-mental-illness-in-ancient-greece-and-rome/282856/

Behere, P.B., Das, A., Yadav, R., & Behere, A.P. (2013). Ayurvedic concepts related to psychotherapy. Indian Journal of Psychiatry, 55(2), 310-314. https://doi.org/10.4103/0019-5545.105556

Casale, S. (2017, December 6). Bedlam: The horrors of London's most notorious insane asylum. The Huffpost. https://www.huffpost.com/entry/bedlam-the-horrors-of-lon_b_9499118

Conrad, L.I., Neve, M., Nutton, V., Porter, R., & and Wear, A. (1995). The western medical tradition 800 BC to AD 1800. Cambridge: Cambridge University Press.

Corrigan, P.W. (2002). Empowerment and serious mental illness: Treatment partnerships and community opportunities. Psychiatric Quarterly, 73(3), 217–228. https://doi.org/10.1023/A:1016040805432

Elkis, H. (2010). History and current definitions of treatment-resistant schizophrenia. Advanced Biological Psychiatry, 26, 1-8. https://doi.org/10.1159/000319805

Fava, G.A., Cosci, F., Guidi, J., & Rafanelli, C. (2020). The deceptive manifestations of treatment resistance in depression: A new look at the problem. Psychotherapy and Psychosomatics, 89(5), 265-273. https://doi.org/10.1159/000507227

Glucklich, A. (2008). The strides of Vishnu: Hindu culture in historical perspective. Oxford University Press.

Kelly, E.B. (2019). Mental illness during the middle ages. Encyclopedia. com. https://www.encyclopedia.com/science/encyclopedias-almanacs-transcripts-and-maps/mental-illness-during-middle-ages

Ruggeri, A. (2016, December 15). How Bedlam became a place for lunatics. BBC. https://www.bbc.com/culture/article/20161213-how-bedlam-became-a-palace-for-lunatics

Schochow, M., & Steger, F. (2013). Johann Christian Reil (1759–1813): Pioneer of psychiatry, city physician, and advocate of public medical care. The American Journal of Psychiatry, 171(4), 403. https://doi.org/10.1176/appi.ajp.2013.13081151

Scull, A. (2014). Cultural sociology of mental illness: An A–Z guide (1st volume). Sage Publications.

Sheitman, B.B., & Lieberman, J.A. (1998). The natural history and pathophysiology of treatment resistant schizophrenia. Journal of Psychiatric Research, 32(3), 143-150. https://doi.org/10.1016/S0022-3956(97)00052-6

Shorter, E (1997). A history of psychiatry: From the era of the asylum to the age of Prozac. John Wiley & Sons, Inc.

Smith, F.M. (2006). The Self Possessed: Deity and Spirit Possession in South Asian Literature and Civilization. Columbia University Press.

Unsworth, C. (1993). Law and lunacy in psychiatry's golden age. Oxford Journal of Legal Studies, 13(4), 476-507. https://doi.org/10.1093/ojls/13.4.479

Chapter 2 References

D'Antonio, P. (2021, May 11). History of psychiatric hospitals. University of Pennsylvania School of Nursing. https://www.nursing.upenn.edu/nhhc/nurses-institutions-caring/history-of-psychiatric-hospitals/.

Demyttenaere, K. (2019). What is treatment resistance in psychiatry? A "difficult to treat" concept. World Psychiatry, 18 (3), 354-255. https://doi.org/10.1002/wps.20677.

Fakhoury, W., and Priebe, S. (2007). Deinstitutionalization and reinstitutionalization: Major changes in the provision of mental healthcare. Psychiatry, 6 (8), 313-316. https://doi.org/10.1016/j.mppsy.2007.05.008.

Fava, G. A., Cosci, F., Guidi, J., and Rafanelli C. (2020). The deceptive manifestations of treatment resistance in depression: A new look at the problem. Psychother Psychosom, 89 (5), 265-273. https://doi.org/10.1159/000507227.

Leckband, S. (2014). Treatment refractory mood disorders: Case report. Mental Health Clinician, 4 (5), 219-220. https://doi.org/10.9740/mhc.n207190.

Lumen Learning. (2021, May 10). Mental health treatment: Then and now. https://courses.lumenlearning.com/wmopen-psychology/chapter/introduction-to-mental-health/.

Roy-Byrne, P. (2015). Treatment-refractory anxiety; definition, risk factors, and treatment challenges. Dialogues Clin Neurosci, 17 (2), 191-206. https://doi.org/10.31887/DCNS.2015.17.2/proybyrne.
Russell, J. B. (1972). Witchcraft in the middle ages. Cornell University Press. Retrieved May 11, 2021, from https://books.google.ca/books?hl=en&lr=&id=LsjagvvkveEC&oi=fnd&pg=PA1&dq=witchcraft&ots=ay6fGo8sNQ&sig=DNxhoBD6e5Q_-9aGRorh5GokXvY&redir_esc=y#v=onepage&q=witchcraft&f=false.

Science Museum. (2018, June 13). A Victorian mental asylum. https://www.sciencemuseum.org.uk/objects-and-stories/medicine/victorian-mental-asylum.

The Time Chamber. (2017, Sept 13). The history of the asylum. https://www.thetimechamber.co.uk/beta/sites/asylums/asylum-history/the-history-of-the-asylum.

Chapter 3 References

Brain, C., Kymes, S., DiBenedetti, D.B., Brevig, T., & Velligan, D.I. (2018). Experiences, attitudes, and perceptions of caregivers of individuals with treatment-resistant schizophrenia: a qualitative study. BMC Psychiatry, 18, 253. https://doi.org/10.1186/s12888-018-1833-5

Correll, C.U., Brevig, T., & Brain, C. (2019). Patient characteristics, burden and pharmacotherapy of treatment-resistant schizophrenia: results from a survey of 204 US psychiatrists. BMC Psychiatry, 19, 362. https://doi.org/10.1186/s12888-019-2318-x

Crown, W. H., Finkelstein, S., Berndt, E. R., Ling, D., Poret, A. W., Rush, A. J., & Russell, J. M. (2002). The impact of treatment-resistant depression on health care utilization and costs.

The Journal of clinical psychiatry, 63(11), 963–971. https://doi.org/10.4088/jcp.v63n1102

Demyttenaere, K., & Van Duppen, Z. (2019). The Impact of (the Concept of)

Treatment-Resistant Depression: An Opinion Review. The international journal of neuropsychopharmacology, 22(2), 85–92. https://doi.org/10.1093/ijnp/pyy052

Fava M. (2003). Diagnosis and definition of treatment-resistant depression. Biological psychiatry, 53(8), 649–659. https://doi.org/10.1016/s0006-3223(03)00231-2

Jaffe, D.H., Rive, B., & Denee, T.R. (2019). The humanistic and economic burden of treatment-resistant depression in Europe: a cross-sectional study. BMC Psychiatry, 19, 247. https://doi.org/10.1186/s12888-019-2222-4

Lepine, B. A., Moreno, R. A., Campos, R. N., & Couttolenc, B. F. (2012). Treatment-resistant depression increases health costs and resource utilization. Revista brasileira de psiquiatria (Sao Paulo, Brazil:1999), 34(4), 379–388. https://doi.org/10.1016/j.rbp.2012.05.009

Mrazek, D.A, Hornberger, J.C., Altar, C.A, & Degtiar, I. (2014). A review of the clinical, economic, and societal burden of treatment-resistant depression: 1996–2013. Psychiatric Services, 65(8), 977–87. https://doi.org/10.1176/appi.ps.201300059.

Treatment-Resistant Conditions. Treatment-Resistant Conditions | Amen Clinics. (n.d.). https://www.amenclinics.com/conditions/treatment-resistant-conditions/.

Chapter 4 References

Barlow, D. H., Gorman, J. M., Katherine Shear, M., & Woods, S. W. (2020). Cognitive-behavioral therapy, imipramine, or their combination for panic disorder: A randomized controlled trial. The Neurotic Paradox, Volume 1: Progress in Understanding and Treating Anxiety and Related Disorders, 283(19), 125–140. https://doi.org/10.4324/9781315724539-11

Bhui, K. (2017). Treatment resistant mental illnesses. British Journal of Psychiatry, 210(6), 443–444. https://doi.org/10.1192/bjp.210.6.443

Bystritsky, A. (2006). Treatment-resistant anxiety disorders. Molecular Psychiatry, 11(9), 805–814. https://doi.org/10.1038/sj.mp.4001852

Caspi, A., Sugden, K., Moffitt, T. E., Taylor, A., Craig, I. W., Harrington, H. L., McClay, J., Mill, J., Martin, J., Braithwaite, A., & Poulton, R. (2003). Influence of life stress on depression: Moderation by a polymorphism in the 5-HTT gene. Science, 301(5631), 386–389. https://doi.org/10.1126/science.1083968

Crown, W. H., Finkelstein, S., Berndt, E. R., Ling, D., Poret, A. W., Rush, A. J., & Russell, J. M. (2002). The impact of treatment-resistant depression on health care utilization and costs. Journal of Clinical Psychiatry, 63(11), 963–971. https://doi.org/10.4088/JCP.v63n1102

Fornaro, M., & Giosuè, P. (2010). Current Nosology of Treatment Resistant Depression: A Controversy Resistant to Revision. Clinical Practice & Epidemiology in Mental Health, 6(1), 20–24. https://doi.org/10.2174/1745017901006010020

Hirschfeld, R. M. A., & Weissman, M. M. (2002). 70 RISK FACTORS FOR MAJOR DEPRESSION AND BIPOLAR DISORDER ROBERT M.A. HIRSCHFELD MYRN AM.

Ivanova, J. I., Birnbaum, H. G., Kidolezi, Y., Subramanian, G., Khan, S. A., & Stensland, M. D. (2010). Direct and indirect costs of employees with treatment-resistant and non-treatment-resistant major depressive disorder. Current Medical Research and Opinion, 26(10), 2475–2484. https://doi.org/10.1185/03007995.2010.517716

Karg, K., Burmeister, M., Shedden, K., & Sen, S. (2011). The serotonin transporter promoter variant (5-HTTLPR), stress, and depression meta-analysis revisited: Evidence of genetic moderation. Archives of General Psychiatry, 68(5), 444–454. https://doi.org/10.1001/archgenpsychiatry.2010.189

Katon, W. (1986). Panic disorder: epidemiology, diagnosis, and treatment in primary care. Undefined.

Kendler, K. S., Bulik, C. M., Silberg, J., Hettema, J. M., Myers, J., & Prescott, C. A. (2000). Childhood sexual abuse and adult psychiatric and substance use disorders in women: An epidemiological and cotwin control analysis. Archives of General Psychiatry, 57(10), 953–959. https://doi.org/10.1001/archpsyc.57.10.953

Klein, E. (2002). The Role of Extended-Release Benzodiazepines in the Treatment of Anxiety: A Risk-Benefit Evaluation With a Focus on Extended-Release Alprazolam. In The Journal of Clinical Psychiatry (Vol. 63, Issue suppl 14). Physicians Postgraduate Press, Inc. https://www.psychiatrist.com/jcp/anxiety/anxiolytics/role-extended-release-benzodiazepines-treatment-anxiety

Kubitz, N., Mehra, M., Potluri, R. C., Garg, N., & Cossrow, N. (2013). Characterization of Treatment Resistant Depression Episodes in a Cohort of Patients from a US Commercial Claims Database. PLoS ONE, 8(10), 1–9. https://doi.org/10.1371/journal.pone.0076882

Lally, J., Ajnakina, O., Di Forti, M., Trotta, A., Demjaha, A., Kolliakou, A., Mondelli, V., Reis Marques, T., Pariante, C., Dazzan, P., Shergil, S. S., Howes, O. D., David, A. S., MacCabe, J. H., Gaughran, F., & Murray,

R. M. (2016). Two distinct patterns of treatment resistance: Clinical predictors of treatment resistance in first-episode schizophrenia spectrum psychoses. Psychological Medicine, 46(15), 3231–3240. https://doi.org/10.1017/S0033291716002014

Legge, S. E., Dennison, C. A., Pardiñas, A. F., Rees, E., Lynham, A. J., Hopkins, L., Bates, L., Kirov, G., Owen, M. J., O'Donovan, M. C., & Walters, J. T. R. (2020). Clinical indicators of treatment-resistant psychosis. British Journal of Psychiatry, 216(5), 259–266. https://doi.org/10.1192/bjp.2019.120

Leucht, S., Corves, C., Arbter, D., Engel, R. R., Li, C., & Davis, J. M. (2009). Second-generation versus first-generation antipsychotic drugs for schizophrenia: a meta-analysis. The Lancet, 373(9657), 31–41. https://doi.org/10.1016/S0140-6736(08)61764-X

Meltzer, H. Y., Rabinowitz, J., Lee, M. A., Cola, P. A., Ranjan, R., Findling, R. L., & Thompson, P. A. (1997). Age at onset and gender of schizophrenic patients in relation to neuroleptic resistance. American Journal of Psychiatry, 154(4), 475–482. https://doi.org/10.1176/ajp.154.4.475

Nemeroff, C. B. (2007). Prevalence and management of treatment-resistant depression. Journal of Clinical Psychiatry, 68(SUPPL. 8), 17–25. https://doi.org/10.4088/JCP.0707e17

Pandarakalam, J. P. (2018). Challenges of treatment-resistant depression. Psychiatria Danubina, 30(3), 273–284. https://doi.org/10.24869/psyd.2018.273

Plakun, E. (2012). and Psychodynamic Psychiatry : Concepts Psychiatry Needs from Psychoanalysis. 40(1), 183–209.

Rizvi, S. J., Donovan, M., Giacobbe, P., Placenza, F., Rotzinger, S., & Kennedy, S. H. (2011). International Review of Psychiatry Neurostimulation therapies for treatment resistant depression: A focus on vagus nerve stimulation and deep brain stimulation. https://doi.org/10.3109/09540261.2011.630993

Rizvi, S. J., Grima, E., Tan, M., Rotzinger, S., Lin, P., McIntyre, R. S., & Kennedy, S. H. (2014). Treatment-resistant depression in primary care across Canada. Canadian Journal of Psychiatry, 59(7), 349–357. https://doi.org/10.1177/070674371405900702

Roy-Byrne, P., Stein, M., Bystrisky, A., & Katon, W. (1998). Pharmacotherapy of panic disorder: Proposed guidelines for the family physician. Journal of the American Board of Family Practice, 11(4), 282–290. https://doi.org/10.3122/jabfm.11.4.282

Shelton, R. C., Osuntokun, O., Heinloth, A. N., & Corya, S. A. (2010). Therapeutic options for treatment-resistant depression. In CNS Drugs (Vol. 24, Issue 2, pp. 131–161). CNS Drugs. https://doi.org/10.2165/11530280-000000000-00000

Souery, D., Amsterdam, J., De Montigny, C., Lecrubier, Y., Montgomery, S., Lipp, O., Racagni, G., Zohar, J., & Mendlewicz, J. (1999). Treatment resistant depression: Methodological overview and operational criteria. European Neuropsychopharmacology, 9(1–2), 83–91. https://doi.org/10.1016/S0924-977X(98)00004-2

Souery, Daniel, Papakostas, G. I., & Trivedi, M. H. (2006). Treatment-Resistant Depression. In The Journal of Clinical Psychiatry (Vol. 67, Issue suppl 6). Physicians Postgraduate Press, Inc. https://www.psychiatrist.com/jcp/depression/treatment-resistant-depression

Unützer, J., & Park, M. (2012). Older adults with severe, treatment-resistant depression. JAMA - Journal of the American Medical Association, 308(9), 909–918. https://doi.org/10.1001/2012.jama.10690

Chapter 5 References

5 Surprising Mental Health Statistics. Mental Health First Aid. (2019). Retrieved 14 May 2021, from https://www.mentalhealthfirstaid.org/2019/02/5-surprising-mental-health-statistics/#:~:text=5%20percent%20of%20adults%20(18,percent%20have%20three%20or%20more.

American Psychiatric Association. (2013). Diagnostic and Statistical Manual of Mental Disorders (5th ed.).

APA Dictionary of Psychology. Dictionary.apa.org. Retrieved 12 May 2021, from https://dictionary.apa.org/treatment-resistance.

Bosely, S. (2018). The drugs do work: antidepressants are effective, study shows. The Guardian. Retrieved 12 May 2021, from https://www.theguardian.com/science/2018/feb/21/the-drugs-do-work-antidepressants-are-effective-study-shows.

Brown, S., Rittenbach, K., Cheung, S., McKean, G., MacMaster, F., & Clement, F. (2019). Current and Common Definitions of Treatment-Resistant Depression: Findings from a Systematic Review and Qualitative Interviews. The Canadian Journal Of Psychiatry, 64(6), 380-387. https://doi.org/10.1177/0706743719828965

Burns, D. (2017). When Helping Doesn't Help. Psychotherapynetworker.org. Retrieved 12 May 2021, from https://www.psychotherapynetworker.org/magazine/article/1076/when-helping-doesnt-help.

Burton, N., & Davison, P. (2012). Living with schizophrenia (2nd ed.). Acheron.

Causes of Treatment-Resistant Depression. WebMD. (2020). Retrieved 12 May 2021, from https://www.webmd.com/depression/treatment-resistant-depression-causes-treatment-resistant-depression

Chou, I., Kuo, C., Huang, Y., Grainge, M., Valdes, A., & See, L. et al. (2016). Familial Aggregation and Heritability of Schizophrenia and Co-aggregation of Psychiatric Illnesses in Affected Families. Schizophrenia Bulletin, 43(5), 1070-1078. https://doi.org/10.1093/schbul/sbw159

Chouinard, G., Jones, B., & Annable, L. (1978). Neuroleptic-induced supersensitivity psychosis. American Journal Of Psychiatry, 135(11), 1409-1410. https://doi.org/10.1176/ajp.135.11.1409

Davis, K. (2017). LSD: Effects and hazards. Medicalnewstoday.com. Retrieved 12 May 2021, from https://www.medicalnewstoday.com/articles/295966.

de Maat, S., de Jonghe, F., Schoevers, R., & Dekker, J. (2009). The Effectiveness of Long-Term Psychoanalytic Therapy: A Systematic Review of Empirical Studies. Harvard Review Of Psychiatry, 17(1), 1-23. https://doi.org/10.1080/10673220902742476

Demjaha, A., Egerton, A., Murray, R., Kapur, S., Howes, O., Stone, J., & McGuire, P. (2014). Antipsychotic Treatment Resistance in Schizophrenia Associated with Elevated Glutamate Levels but Normal Dopamine Function. Biological Psychiatry, 75(5), e11-e13. https://doi.org/10.1016/j.biopsych.2013.06.011

Demyttenaere, K. (2019). What is treatment resistance in psychiatry? A "difficult to treat" concept. World Psychiatry, 18(3), 354-355. https://doi.org/10.1002/wps.20677

Douaihy, A., Kelly, T., & Sullivan, C. (2013). Medications for Substance Use Disorders. Social Work In Public Health, 28(3-4), 264-278. https://doi.org/10.1080/19371918.2013.759031

Drugs, Brains, and Behaviour: The Science of Addiction. National Institute on Drug Abuse. (2020). Retrieved 14 May 2021, from https://www.drugabuse.gov/publications/drugs-brains-behavior-science-addiction/drugs-brain.

Dryden-Edwards, R. (2017). What Is the Chemical Imbalance that Causes Schizophrenia?. MedicineNet. Retrieved 12 May 2021, from https://www.medicinenet.com/chemical_imbalance_causes_schizophrenia/ask.htm.

Ducci, F., & Goldman, D. (2012). The Genetic Basis of Addictive Disorders. Psychiatric Clinics Of North America, 35(2), 495-519. https://doi.org/10.1016/j.psc.2012.03.010

Eisenberg, D., & Lipson, S. (2019). The Healthy Minds Study. Healthymindsnetwork.org. Retrieved 12 May 2021, from https://healthymindsnetwork.org/wp-content/uploads/2019/09/HMS_national-2018-19.pdf.

Fava, M. (2003). Diagnosis and definition of treatment-resistant depression. Biological Psychiatry, 53(8), 649-659. https://doi.org/10.1016/s0006-3223(03)00231-2

Grover, S., Gautam, S., Jain, A., Gautam, M., & Vahia, V. (2017). Clinical Practice Guidelines for the Management of Depression. Indian Journal Of Psychiatry, 59(5), 34. https://doi.org/10.4103/0019-5545.196973

James, S., Abate, D., Abate, K., Abay, S., Abbafati, C., & Abbasi, N. et al. (2018). Global, regional, and national incidence, prevalence, and years lived with disability for 354 diseases and injuries for 195 countries and territories, 1990-2017: a systematic analysis for the Global Burden of Disease Study 2017. The Lancet, 392(10159), 1789-1858. https://doi.org/10.1016/s0140-6736(18)32279-7

Kabisa, E., Biracyaza, E., Habagusenga, J., & Umubyeyi, A. (2021). Determinants and prevalence of relapse among patients with substance use disorders: case of Icyizere Psychotherapeutic Centre. Substance Abuse Treatment, Prevention, And Policy, 16(1). https://doi.org/10.1186/s13011-021-00347-0

Larsen, R., Buss, D., King, D., & Ensley, C. (2020). Personality Psychology: Domains of Knowledge About Human Nature (2nd ed.). McGraw Hill Education.

Lesser, B. (2021). The Connection Between Mental Illness and Substance Abuse. Dualdiagnosis.org. Retrieved 14 May 2021, from https://dualdiagnosis.org/mental-health-and-addiction/the-connection/.

Li, P., L. Snyder, G., & E. Vanover, K. (2016). Dopamine Targeting Drugs for the Treatment of Schizophrenia: Past, Present and Future. Current Topics In Medicinal Chemistry, 16(29), 3385-3403. https://doi.org/10.2174/1568026616666160608084834

Mental health awareness campaign leads to increase in the number of people seeking help, new CAMH study reveals. CAMH. Retrieved 12 May 2021, from https://www.camh.ca/en/camh-news-and-stories/awareness-campaign-leads-to-increase-in-people-seeking-help.

Mental health. Who.int. Retrieved 12 May 2021, from https://www.who.int/health-topics/mental-health#tab=tab_1.

Morris, J. (2019). Treatment Resistant or Misdiagnosed?. Gwinnett Citizen Newspaper. Retrieved 14 May 2021, from https://gwinnettcitizen.com/health-wellness/eastside-physician-s-spotlight/4687-treatment-resistant-or-misdiagnosed.

Mufson, L. (1999). Efficacy of Interpersonal Psychotherapy for Depressed Adolescents. Archives Of General Psychiatry, 56(6), 573-579. https://doi.org/10.1001/archpsyc.56.6.573

National Institute on Drug Abuse. (2020). Part 1: The Connection Between Substance Use Disorders and Mental Illness. NIDA. Retrieved from https://www.drugabuse.gov/publications/research-reports/common-comorbidities-substance-use-disorders/part-1-connection-between-substance-use-disorders-mental-illness

Oaklander, M. (2017). New Hope for Depression. TIME.com. Retrieved 16 May 2021, from https://time.com/magazine/us/4876068/august-7th-2017-vol-190-no-6-u-s/.

Paparelli, A., Di Forti, M., Morrison, P., & Murray, R. (2011). Drug-Induced Psychosis: How to Avoid Star Gazing in Schizophrenia Research by Looking at More Obvious Sources of Light. Frontiers In Behavioral Neuroscience, 5. https://doi.org/10.3389/fnbeh.2011.00001
Patel, K., Cherian, J., Gohil, K., & Atkinson, D. (2014). Schizophrenia: Overview and Treatment Options. P & T : A Peer-Reviewed Journal For Formulary Management, 39(9), 638-45. Retrieved 12 May 2021, from.

Potenza, M. (2013). Biological Contributions to Addictions in Adolescents and Adults: Prevention, Treatment, and Policy Implications. Journal Of Adolescent Health, 52(2), S22-S32. https://doi.org/10.1016/j.jadohealth.2012.05.007

Potkin, S., Kane, J., Correll, C., Lindenmayer, J., Agid, O., & Marder, S. et al. (2020). The neurobiology of treatment-resistant schizophrenia: paths to antipsychotic resistance and a roadmap for future research. Npj Schizophrenia, 6(1). https://doi.org/10.1038/s41537-019-0090-z

Principles of Effective Treatment. National Institute on Drug Abuse. (2018). Retrieved 14 May 2021, from https://www.drugabuse.gov/publications/principles-drug-addiction-treatment-research-based-guide-third-edition/principles-effective-treatment.

Pun, J. (2019). What is Online Cognitive Behavioral Therapy (CBT)? - Starling Minds | Starling Minds. Starling Minds. Retrieved 12 May 2021, from https://www.starlingminds.com/what-is-online-cognitive-behavioral-therapy-cbt-starling-minds/#:~:text=CBT%20alone%20is%2050%2D75,helping%20people%20overcome%20mental%20illness.

Rennie, D. (1994). Clients' deference in psychotherapy. Journal Of Counseling Psychology, 41(4), 427-437. https://doi.org/10.1037/0022-0167.41.4.427

Shaffer, H. (2017). What is addiction? - Harvard Health. Harvard Health. Retrieved 14 May 2021, from https://www.health.harvard.edu/blog/what-is-addiction-2-2017061914490.

Sinclair, D., Zhao, S., Qi, F., Nyakyoma, K., Kwong, J., & Adams, C. (2019). Electroconvulsive Therapy for Treatment-Resistant Schizophrenia. Schizophrenia Bulletin, 45(4), 730-732. https://doi.org/10.1093/schbul/sbz037

Spooner, C., & Hetherington, K. (2004). SOCIAL DETERMINANTS OF DRUG USE (pp. 79-160). Sydney: NATIONAL DRUG AND ALCOHOL RESEARCH CENTRE, UNIVERSITY OF NEW SOUTH WALES.

Stangier, U. (2011). Cognitive Therapy vs Interpersonal Psychotherapy in Social Anxiety Disorder. Archives Of General Psychiatry, 68(7), 692. https://doi.org/10.1001/archgenpsychiatry.2011.67

Treatment and Recovery. National Institute on Drug Abuse. (2018). Retrieved 14 May 2021, from https://www.drugabuse.gov/publications/drugs-brains-behavior-science-addiction/treatment-recovery.

Treatment-Resistant Conditions. Amenclinics.com. Retrieved 14 May 2021, from https://www.amenclinics.com/conditions/treatment-resistant-conditions/.

van Hees, M., Rotter, T., Ellermann, T., & Evers, S. (2013). The effectiveness of individual interpersonal psychotherapy as a treatment for major depressive disorder in adult outpatients: a systematic review. BMC Psychiatry, 13(1). https://doi.org/10.1186/1471-244x-13-22

What Is Depression?. Psychiatry.org. (2020). Retrieved 12 May 2021, from https://www.psychiatry.org/patients-families/depression/what-is-depression.

What Is Schizophrenia?. Psychiatry.org. Retrieved 12 May 2021, from https://www.psychiatry.org/patients-families/schizophrenia/what-is-schizophrenia.

Why Antidepressants Don't Work For So Many. ScienceDaily. (2009). Retrieved 12 May 2021, from https://www.sciencedaily.com/releases/2009/10/091023163346.htm.

Zaheer, J., Olfson, M., Mallia, E., Lam, J., de Oliveira, C., & Rudoler, D. et al. (2020). Predictors of suicide at time of diagnosis in schizophrenia spectrum disorder: A 20-year total population study in Ontario, Canada. Schizophrenia Research, 222, 382-388. https://doi.org/10.1016/j.schres.2020.04.025

Chapter 6 References

Amen Clinics. (2021). Treatment-Resistant Conditions. Amen Clinics. https://www.amenclinics.com/conditions/treatment-resistant-conditions/

Brenner, P., Brandt, L., Li, G., DiBernardo, A., Bodén, R., & Reutfors, J. (2020). Substance use disorders and risk for treatment resistant depression: a population-based, nested case-control study. Addiction, 115(4), 768–777. https://doi-org.login.ezproxy.library.ualberta.ca/10.1111/add.14866

Bystritsky, A. (2006). Treatment-resistant anxiety disorders. Molecular Psychiatry, 11(9), 805–814. https://doi-org.login.ezproxy.library.ualberta.ca/10.1038/sj.mp.4001852

Casetta, C., Montrasio, C., Cheli, S., Baldelli, S., Bianchi, I., Clementi,

E., Gambini, O., & D'Agostino, A. (2019). Pharmacogenetic variants in bipolar disorder with elevated treatment resistance and intolerance: Towards a personalized pattern of care. Bipolar Disorders, 21(3), 288–291. https://doi-org.login.ezproxy.library.ualberta.ca/10.1111/bdi.12763

Cepeda, M. S., Reps, J., Fife, D., Blacketer, C., Stang, P., & Ryan, P. (2018). Finding treatment-resistant depression in real-world data: How a data-driven approach compares with expert-based heuristics. Depression and Anxiety, 35(3), 220–228. https://doi-org.login.ezproxy.library.ualberta.ca/10.1002/da.22705

Friedman, L. M., McBurnett, K., Dvorsky, M. R., Hinshaw, S. P., & Pfiffner, L. J. (2020). Learning Disorder Confers Setting-Specific Treatment Resistance for Children with ADHD, Predominantly Inattentive Presentation. Journal of Clinical Child & Adolescent Psychology, 49(6), 854–867. https://doi-org.login.ezproxy.library.ualberta.ca/10.1080/15374416.2019.1644647

Michele Fornaro, Andrea Fusco, Stefano Novello, Pierluigi Mosca, Annalisa Anastasia, Antonella De Blasio, Felice Iasevoli, & Andrea de Bartolomeis. (2020). Predictors of Treatment Resistance Across Different Clinical Subtypes of Depression: Comparison of Unipolar vs. Bipolar Cases. Frontiers in Psychiatry, 11. https://doi-org.login.ezproxy.library.ualberta.ca/10.3389/fpsyt.2020.00438

Morup, M. F., Kymes, S. M., & Oudin Astrom, D. (2020). A modelling approach to estimate the prevalence of treatment-resistant schizophrenia in the United States. PLoS ONE, 15(6), 1–10. https://doi.org/10.1371/journal/pone/0234121

Orr-Brown, D. E., & Siebert, D. C. (2007). Resistance in Adolescent Substance Abuse Treatment: A Literature Synthesis. Journal of Social Work Practice in the Addictions, 7(3), 5–28. https://doi-org.login.ezproxy.library.ualberta.ca/10.1300/J160v07n03_02

Shearer, R. A., & Ogan, G. D. (2002). Voluntary Participation and Treatment Resistance in Substance Abuse Treatment Programs. Journal of Offender Rehabilitation, 34(3), 31. https://doi-org.login.ezproxy.library.ualberta.ca/10.1300/J076v34n03_03

Sternat T, Fotinos K, Fine A, Epstein I, & Katzman MA. (2018). Low hedonic tone and attention-deficit hyperactivity disorder: risk factors for treatment resistance in depressed adults. Neuropsychiatric Disease and Treatment, ume 14, 2379–2387.

Chapter 7 References

Brisch, R., Saniotis, A., Wolf, R., Bielau, H., Bernstein, H. G., Steiner, J., Bogerts, B., Braun, K., Jankowski, Z., Kumaratilake, J., Henneberg, M., & Gos, T. (2014). The role of dopamine in schizophrenia from a neurobiological and evolutionary perspective: old fashioned, but still in vogue. Frontiers in psychiatry, 5, 47. https://doi.org/10.3389/fpsyt.2014.00047

F. Caraci, F. Calabrese, R. Molteni, L. Bartova, M. Dold, G. M. Leggio, C. Fabbri, J. Mendlewicz, G. Racagni, S. Kasper, M. A. Riva and F. Drago Pharmacological Reviews July 1, 2018, 70 (3) 475-504; DOI: https://doi.org/10.1124/pr.117.014977

Nesrin Dilbaz, Serçin Yalcın Cavus and Aslı Enez Darcin (September 12th 2011). Treatment Resistant Generalized Anxiety Disorder, Different Views of Anxiety Disorders, Salih Selek, IntechOpen, DOI: 10.5772/23255.

Demyttenaere, K. (2019). What is treatment resistance in psychiatry? A "difficult to treat" concept. World Psychiatry, 18(3), 354–355. https://doi.org/10.1002/wps.20677

Etkin, A., Maron-Katz, A., Wu, W., Fonzo, G., Huemer, J., Vértes, P., Patenaude, B., Richiardi, J., Goodkind, M., Keller, C., Ramos-Cejudo, J., Zaiko, Y., Peng, K., Shpigel, E., Longwell, P., Toll, R., Thompson, A., Zack, S., Gonzalez, B., ... O'Hara, R. (2019). Using fMRI connectivity to define a treatment-resistant form of post-traumatic stress disorder. Science Translational Medicine, 11(486), eaal3236–. https://doi.org/10.1126/scitranslmed.aal3236

Fabbri, C., Marsano, A., Albani, D., Chierchia, A., Calati, R., Drago, A., ... & Serretti, A. (2014). PPP3CC gene: a putative modulator of antidepressant response through the B-cell receptor signaling pathway. The pharmacogenomics journal, 14(5), 463-472.

Fabbri, C., Corponi, F., Albani, D., Raimondi, I., Forloni, G., Schruers, K., ... & Serretti, A. (2018). Pleiotropic genes in psychiatry: Calcium channels and the stress-related FKBP5 gene in antidepressant resistance. Progress in Neuro-Psychopharmacology and Biological Psychiatry, 81, 203-210.

Iliades, C. (2019, January 28). Approaching Treatment-Resistant Anxiety. Psychiatry Advisor. https://www.psychiatryadvisor.com/home/topics/anxiety/approaching-treatment-resistant-anxiety/3/.

Martin, E. I., Ressler, K. J., Binder, E., & Nemeroff, C. B. (2009). The neurobiology of anxiety disorders: brain imaging, genetics, and psychoneuroendocrinology. The Psychiatric clinics of North America, 32(3), 549–575. https://doi.org/10.1016/j.psc.2009.05.004

Mathew, S. J., Mao, X., Coplan, J. D., Smith, E. L., Sackeim, H. A., Gorman, J. M., & Shungu, D. C. (2004). Dorsolateral prefrontal cortical pathology in generalized anxiety disorder: a proton magnetic resonance spectroscopic imaging study. American Journal of Psychiatry, 161(6), 1119-1121.

Paddock, S., Laje, G., Charney, D., Rush, A. J., Wilson, A. F., Sorant, A. J., ... & McMahon, F. J. (2007). Association of GRIK4 with outcome of antidepressant treatment in the STAR* D cohort. American Journal of Psychiatry, 164(8), 1181-1188

Roy-Byrne P. (2015). Treatment-refractory anxiety; definition, risk factors, and treatment challenges. Dialogues in clinical neuroscience, 17(2), 191–206. https://doi.org/10.31887/DCNS.2015.17.2/proybyrne

Sattar, Y., Wilson, J., Khan, A. M., Adnan, M., Azzopardi Larios, D., Shrestha, S., Rahman, Q., Mansuri, Z., Hassan, A., Patel, N. B., Tariq, N., Latchana, S., Lopez Pantoja, S. C., Vargas, S., Shaikh, N. A., Syed, F., Mittal, D., & Rumesa, F. (2018). A Review of the Mechanism of Antagonism of N-methyl-D-aspartate Receptor by Ketamine in Treatment-resistant Depression. Cureus, 10(5), e2652. https://doi.org/10.7759/cureus.2652

Vanes, L. D., Mouchlianitis, E., Collier, T., Averbeck, B. B., & Shergill, S. S. (2018). Differential neural reward mechanisms in treatment-responsive and treatment-resistant schizophrenia. Psychological medicine, 48(14), 2418–2427. https://doi.org/10.1017/S0033291718000041

Wohleb, E., Franklin, T., Iwata, M. et al. Integrating neuroimmune systems in the neurobiology of depression. Nat Rev Neurosci 17, 497–511 (2016). https://doi.org/10.1038/nrn.2016.69

Whitten, L. A. (2012). Functional magnetic resonance imaging (fMRI): An invaluable tool in translational neuroscience RTI Press Publication No. OP-0010-1212. Research Triangle Park, NC: RTI Press. https://doi.org/10.3768/rtipress.2012.op.0010.1212

Chapter 8 References

Arsalan, A., Iqbal, Z., Tariq, M., Ayonrinde, O., Vincent, J. B., & Ayub, M. (2019). Association of smoked cannabis with treatment resistance in schizophrenia. Psychiatry Research, 278(Complete), 242–247. https://doi.org/10.1016/j.psychres.2019.06.023

Aspen, V., Darcy, A. M., & Lock, J. (2014). Patient Resistance in Eating Disorders. Psychiatric Times. https://www.psychiatrictimes.com/view/patient-resistance-eating-disorders.

Bandelow, B., Michaelis, S., & Wedekind, D. (2017). Treatment of anxiety disorders. Dialogues in clinical neuroscience, 19(2), 93–107. https://doi.org/10.31887/DCNS.2017.19.2/bbandelow

Bennabi, D., Charpeaud, T., Yrondi, A. et al. Clinical guidelines for the management of treatment-resistant depression: French recommendations from experts, the French Association for Biological Psychiatry and Neuropsychopharmacology and the fondation FondaMental. BMC Psychiatry 19, 262 (2019). https://doi.org/10.1186/s12888-019-2237-x

Bystritsky, A. Treatment-resistant anxiety disorders. Mol Psychiatry 11, 805–814 (2006). https://doi.org/10.1038/sj.mp.4001852

Conley, R. R., & Kelly, D. L. (2001). Management of treatment resistance in schizophrenia. Biological Psychiatry, 50(11), 898–911. https://doi.org/10.1016/S0006-3223(01)01271-9

Demyttenaere K. (2019). What is treatment resistance in psychiatry? A "difficult to treat" concept. World psychiatry : official journal of the World Psychiatric Association (WPA), 18(3), 354–355. https://doi.org/10.1002/wps.20677

Facts & Statistics: Anxiety and Depression Association of America, ADAA. Facts & Statistics | Anxiety and Depression Association of America, ADAA. (n.d.). https://adaa.org/understanding-anxiety/facts-statistics.

Fava, M. (2003). Diagnosis and definition of treatment-resistant depression. Biological Psychiatry, 53(8), 649–659. https://doi.org/10.1016/S0006-3223(03)00231-2

Guarda, A. (Ed.). (2021). What Are Eating Disorders? American Psychiatric Association (APA). https://www.psychiatry.org/patients-families/eating-disorders/what-are-eating-disorders.

Halmi, K.A. Perplexities of treatment resistance in eating disorders. BMC Psychiatry 13, 292 (2013). https://doi.org/10.1186/1471-244X-13-292

Lifestyle Changes to Manage Depression. Winchester Hospital. (2020). https://www.winchesterhospital.org/health-library/article?id=19338.

Lopresti, A. L., Hood, S. D., & Drummond, P. D. (2013). A review of lifestyle factors that contribute to important pathways associated with major depression: Diet, sleep and exercise. Journal of Affective Disorders, 148(1), 12–27. https://doi.org/10.1016/j.jad.2013.01.014

Mayo Foundation for Medical Education and Research. (2017, July 14). Eating disorder treatment: Know your options. Mayo Clinic. https://www.mayoclinic.org/diseases-conditions/eating-disorders/in-depth/eating-disorder-treatment/art-20046234.

Mayo Foundation for Medical Education and Research. (2020, January 7). Schizophrenia. Mayo Clinic. https://www.mayoclinic.org/diseases-conditions/schizophrenia/diagnosis-treatment/drc-20354449.

Impact of Eating Disorders on Quality of Life - and How Treatment Centers Can Help. Monte Nido. (2020, November 6). https://www.montenido.com/impact-of-eating-disorders/.

Omudhome Ogbru, P. D. (2018, October 16). 28 Antidepressants Types, Side Effects, List & Alcohol Interactions. MedicineNet. https://www.medicinenet.com/antidepressants/article.htm#what_are_antidepressants_depression_medications.

Potkin, S.G., Kane, J.M., Correll, C.U. et al. The neurobiology of treatment-resistant schizophrenia: paths to antipsychotic resistance and a roadmap for future research. npj Schizophr 6, 1 (2020). https://doi.org/10.1038/s41537-019-0090-z

Press Releases- Facts on Schizophrenia. NAMI. (1998). https://www.nami.org/press-Media/Press-Releases/1998/Facts-on-Schizophrenia#:~:text=Schizophrenia%20is%20a%20brain%20disorder,schizophrenia%2C%20but%20this%20is%20uncommon.

Souery, D., Papakostas, G., & Trivedi, M. H. (2006). Treatment-Resistant Depression. Psychiatrist.com. https://www.psychiatrist.com/wp-content/uploads/2021/02/18423_treatment-resistant-depression.pdf.

The most effective antidepressants for adults revealed in major review. NIHR Evidence. (2021, February 12). https://evidence.nihr.ac.uk/alert/the-most-effective-antidepressants-for-adults-revealed-in-major-review/.

Trivedi, M. H. (2013). Modeling Predictors, Moderators and Mediators of Treatment Outcome and Resistance in Depression. Biological Psychiatry, 74(1), 2–4. https://doi.org/10.1016/j.biopsych.2013.05.009 WebMD. (2020). Generalized Anxiety Disorder Treatment & Medications. WebMD. https://www.webmd.com/anxiety-panic/guide/understanding-anxiety-treatment.

Weiden, P. J. (2016). How Many Treatments Before Clozapine?

Medication Choices Across the Spectrum of Treatment Resistance in Schizophrenia. Psychiatrist.com. https://www-psychiatrist-com. proxy.library.brocku.ca/jcp/schizophrenia/many-treatments-before-clozapine-medication-choices/.

Chapter 9 References

Chopra, A. K. (2020). Metabolic Syndrome or Insulin Resistance: Evolution, Controversies and Association With Cardiovascular Disease Risk. Indian Journal of Clinical Cardiology, 1(2), 77–85. https://doi. org/10.1177/2632463620935030

Fornaro, M., & Giosuè, P. (2010). Current nosology of treatment resistant depression: a controversy resistant to revision. Clinical practice and epidemiology in mental health : CP & EMH, 6, 20–24. https://doi.org/10.2174/1745017901006010020

Gitlin, M. Treatment-resistant bipolar disorder. Mol Psychiatry 11, 227–240 (2006). https://doi.org/10.1038/sj.mp.4001793

Slowiczek, L. (2019, May 25). Spravato: Uses, side effects, dosage, and more. Medical News Today. https://www.medicalnewstoday.com/articles/326038#alternatives.

Staudt, M. D., Herring, E. Z., Gao, K., Miller, J. P., & Sweet, J. A. (2019). Evolution in the Treatment of Psychiatric Disorders: From Psychosurgery to Psychopharmacology to Neuromodulation. Frontiers in neuroscience, 13, 108. https://doi.org/10.3389/fnins.2019.00108

Tilles, G., Wallach, D., & Taïeb, A. (2007). Topical therapy of atopic dermatitis: controversies from Hippocrates to topical immunomodulators. Journal of the American Academy of Dermatology, 56(2), 295–301. https://doi.org/10.1016/j.jaad.2006.09.030

Chapter 10 References

Al-Harbi, K. S. (2012). Treatment-resistant depression: therapeutic trends, challenges, and future directions. Patient preference and adherence. https://www.ncbi.nlm.nih.gov/pmc/articles/PMC3363299/.

www.ingramcontent.com/pod-product-compliance
Lightning Source LLC
Chambersburg PA
CBHW021823190326
41518CB00007B/723